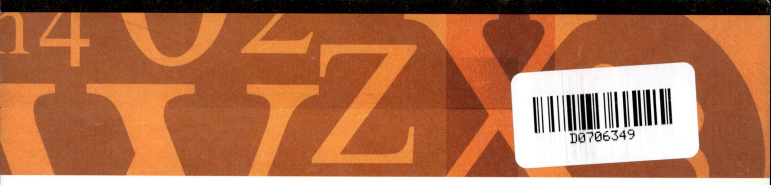

MediSoft Made Easy
A Step-by-Step Approach
Second Edition

Lori Tyler, BA, MS

Lillian D. Burke, AAS, BBA, MA
Middlesex County College

Barbara Weill, BA, MA, PhD, AA
Middlesex County College

Pearson

Boston   Columbus   Indianapolis   New York   San Francisco   Upper Saddle River
Amsterdam   Cape Town   Dubai   London   Madrid   Milan   Munich   Paris
Montreal   Toronto   Delhi   Mexico City   São Paulo   Sydney
Hong Kong   Seoul   Singapore   Taipei   Tokyo

Library of Congress Cataloging-in-Publication Data

Tyler, Lori.
    MediSoft made easy: a step-by-step approach/Lori Tyler, Lillian Burke, Barbara Weill.—2nd ed.
        p. cm.
    Includes index.
    ISBN-13: 978-0-13-813139-5
    ISBN-10: 0-13-813139-2
1. MediSoft. 2. Medical informatics. 3. Medical offices—Automation. I. Burke, Lillian. II. Weill, Barbara.
III. Title.
    [DNLM: 1. MediSoft. 2. Office Automation—Programmed Instruction. 3. Practice Management—Programmed
Instruction. 4. Software—Programmed Instruction. W 18.2 T982m 2011]
    R858.B856 2011
    651′.9610285–dc22

                                                                                                2009015741

Publisher: Julie Levin Alexander
Publisher's Assistant: Regina Bruno
Editor-in-Chief: Mark Cohen
Executive Editor: Joan Gill
Associate Editor: Bronwen Glowacki
Editorial Assistant: Mary Ellen Ruitenberg
Director of Marketing: Karen Allman
Senior Marketing Manager: Harper Coles
Marketing Specialist: Michael Sirinides
Marketing Assistant: Judy Noh
Managing Production Editor: Patrick Walsh
Production Liaison: Julie Boddorf
Production Editor: Ravi Bhatt
Senior Media Editor: Amy Peltier
Media Project Manager: Lorena Cerisano
Manufacturing Manager: Ilene Sanford

Manufacturing Buyer: Pat Brown
Creative Director: Jayne Conte
Senior Art Director: Maria Guglielmo
Art Director: Kristine Carney
Interior Designer: Dina Curro
Cover Designer: Dina Curro
Cover Image: istockphoto
Director, Image Resource Center: Melinda Reo
Manager, Rights and Permissions: Zina Arabia
Manager, Visual Research: Beth Brenzel
Manager, Cover Visual Research and Permissions:
    Karen Sanatar
Image Permission Coordinator: Kathy Gavilanes
Composition: Aptara®, Inc.
Printing and Binding: Courier Kendallville
Cover Printer: Lehigh-Phoenix Color

MediSoft is a registered trademark of NDC Health.

Screenshots used by permission of MCKESSON Corporation. All rights reserved. © MCKESSON Corporation 2007.

Notice: The author and the publisher of this volume have taken care that the information and technical recommendations contained herein are based on research and expert consultation, and are accurate and compatible with the standards generally accepted at the time of publication. Nevertheless, as new information becomes available, changes in clinical and technical practices become necessary. The reader is advised to carefully consult manufacturers' instructions and information material for all supplies and equipment before use and to consult with a health care professional as necessary. This advice is especially important when using new supplies or equipment for clinical purposes. The author and publisher disclaim all responsibility for any liability, loss, injury, or damage incurred as a consequence, directly or indirectly, of the use and application of any of the contents of this volume.

10 9 8 7 6 5 4 3 2 1

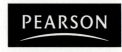

www.pearsonhighered.com

ISBN 13: 978-0-13-813139-5
ISBN 10:   0-13-813139-2

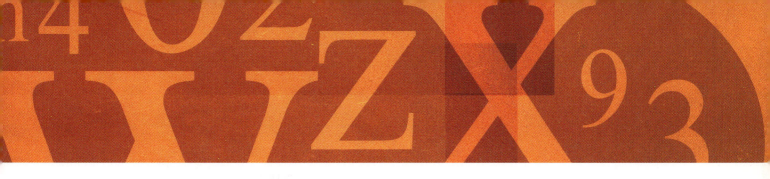

BRIEF CONTENTS

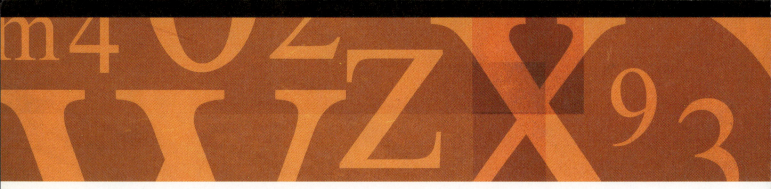

CONTENTS

PREFACE

Computer technology is transforming all aspects of our lives, including how we think, analyze, educate, buy, protect, and care for one another. The term *medical informatics* refers to the use of computer technology in health care and its delivery. The skillful use of computers and software programs is the key to success in virtually all of today's professions. This is particularly true in health care fields, where students, health care providers, and office personnel need to use computer technology. MediSoft computer software can help computerize administrative functions in the medical office, including entering and editing patient, provider, and case information; entering and editing transaction charges, payments, and adjustment information; creating and managing claims; and creating and printing various kinds of reports. All this information is saved in tables in a relational database (an organized collection of related data). *MediSoft Made Easy* is geared toward the medical office worker and student of medical office administration.

The first chapter of *MediSoft Made Easy* is a general introduction to medical informatics. Chapter 2 familiarizes the reader with the Windows environment and basic Windows terminology. Chapter 3 is an overview of using MediSoft in the medical office. It should be noted that some examples in this book take place in an unrealistic time frame. For example, in Chapter 10, the discussion assumes the insurer pays a claim the same day a patient is seen; this would never happen.

Chapters 4–11 are a step-by-step hands-on introduction to MediSoft. We approached MediSoft as novice users would approach it, and presented it to the student in the same fashion. In Chapter 4, the reader learns how to make appointments using MediSoft's scheduling software, the Appointment Book. In Chapter 5, the reader learns how to enter patient and case information. Chapters 6 and 7 introduce the reader to entering transactions and processing claims. In Chapters 8 and 9, the reader learns how to print and design reports. In Chapter 10, we review all the previous tasks by taking the student through the process of creating a new database for a new practice. Some tasks, such as using MediSoft utilities, cannot be performed in a classroom setting. However, these aspects of the program are covered in Chapter 11 so the student has at least some familiarity with them in a real working environment.

New to MediSoft version 14 is the capability of completing UB-04 Claims using MediSoft. Appendix 1 teaches students how to use this function. Appendix 2 is recommended for students who have no knowledge of computers. It introduces the student to computers and computer literacy, including basic computer terminology.

We would like to thank the following people for reviewing this book in manuscript form: Ramona Atiles, LPN, RPT, CET, Allied Health Program Coordinator, Career Institute of Health and Technology, Garden City, NY; Donna Kyle-Brown, RMA, CPC, Educational Coordinator/Medical Billing and Coding Program, Virginia College Gulf Coast, Biloxi, MS; Rebecca Croom, Program Director, Virginia College, Huntsville, AL; Marie Crow; CPC, CCS-P, Department Chairperson, St. Louis College of Health Careers, St. Louis, MO; Gloria J. Hoover, CMA (AAMA), AAS, Faculty, Central Piedmont Community College, Charlotte, NC; Belinda Sasala, BS Education, Faculty Development and Registrar, Bohecker College, Ravenna, OH; Mary Warren-Oliver, BS, Medical Program Chair, Sanford-Brown College, Vienna, VA; Mindy Wray, BS, CMA, RMA, Health Sciences Department Head, ECPI College of Technology, Jamestown, NC.

Lori Tyler

CHAPTER ONE

AN INTRODUCTION TO MEDICAL INFORMATICS

Chapter Outline

- Medical Informatics
- Administrative Applications of Computer Technology in the Medical Office Using MediSoft
- Clinical Applications
- Special-Purpose Applications
- Telemedicine
- Privacy and Security of Medical Information
- The Health Insurance Portability and Accountability Act of 1996
- Summary
- Review Exercises

Learning Objectives

Upon completion of this chapter, the student will be able to:

- Define medical informatics.
- Define clinical, special-purpose, and administrative applications of computer technology in health care and its delivery.
- Define telemedicine.
- Define administrative applications of computer technology in health care, with specific reference to MediSoft.
- Discuss issues related to the privacy and security of medical information.
- Explain the privacy protections of the Health Insurance Portability and Accountability Act.

Key Terms

Administrative Application

Balance Billing

Biometric

Bucket Billing

Callback Systems

Clinical Application

Computerized Tomography (CT) scan

Decryption

Electronic Medical Record (EMR)

Encryption

Expert Systems

Firewall

Health Insurance Portability and Accountability Act (HIPAA)

Human Genome Project

Magnetic Resonance Imaging (MRI)

Medical Informatics

MediSoft

PIN (Personal Identification
   Number)

Positron-Emission
   Tomography (PET) Scan

Protected Health Information
   (PHI)

Relational Database

Special-Purpose Application

Telemedicine

Medical Informatics

The use of computers and computer information technology in health care and its delivery is called **medical informatics**. Traditionally, the application of computer technology in health care is divided into three categories:

1. The **clinical applications** of computers include anything that has to do with direct patient care, including diagnosis, treatment, and monitoring.
2. **Special-purpose applications** include the use of computers in teaching and some aspects of pharmacy.
3. **Administrative applications** include office management, scheduling, and billing tasks. MediSoft and other programs like it are specifically designed for medical office management.

   Telemedicine—the delivery of health care over telecommunication lines—crosses all traditional boundaries and includes clinical, special-purpose, and administrative applications.
   Beginning with the computerization of hospital administrative tasks in the 1960s, the role of digital technology in medical care and its delivery has expanded at an ever-increasing pace. Today computers play a part in every aspect of health care.

Administrative Applications of Computer Technology in the Medical Office Using MediSoft

As stated, administrative applications include office management tasks, scheduling, and billing. These are tasks that need to be performed in any office. However, some of these activities are slightly different in a health-care environment, so programs that address the special needs of a medical office are needed.
   MediSoft is a program specifically designed to computerize basic administrative functions in a health-care environment. It allows the user to organize information by patient, case, and provider. The user can schedule patient appointments; take electronic progress notes; create lists of codes for diagnosis, treatment, and insurance; submit claims to insurers; and receive payments electronically. MediSoft is capable of working with the **bucket billing**, or **balance billing**, that medical offices must use to bill two or three insurers in a timely fashion *before* the patient is billed. Moreover, because MediSoft is a **relational database** (an organized collection of related data), information input in one part of the program can be linked to information in another part of the program, avoiding the need to input data more than once. Billing information and financial status are easily available in MediSoft. Data can be presented in finished form in one of the many report designs provided, including various kinds of billing reports. If there is not a report design that meets the user's need, a customized report can easily be designed and generated by the user.

Clinical Applications

In addition to computer software programs such as MediSoft that are used primarily in medical office settings, other computer programs and technology are used in hospital environments. Nurses and staff can oversee patient care from centrally located cameras and monitoring stations that provide instant access to a patient's condition. For help with diagnosis, sophisticated digital imaging techniques, including **computerized tomography (CT) scans**, **magnetic resonance imaging (MRI)**, and **positron emission tomography (PET) scans**, are supplementing the use of x-rays as digital images replace film images. **Expert systems**, which turn the computer into an expert in one specific area, can help medical personnel diagnose and treat conditions they have never seen. There are many expert systems in medicine: POEMS, for example, deals specifically with postoperative complications. INTERNIST is an expert on bacterial infections. Robotic devices take part in surgeries. ROBODOC drills the hole in the femur for cementless hip replacements. AESOP holds the endoscope in laparoscopic surgeries. DaVinci has performed long-distance surgeries; for example, a patient in Bosnia was operated on by a robot controlled by a doctor in Germany.

The microprocessor, a computer on a chip of silicon, which is embedded in many home appliances, is also embedded in many medical appliances such as defibrillators, IV (intravenous) pumps, incubators, and heart pacemakers. What makes a microprocessor-controlled device unique is that, like larger computers, it can be programmed and respond to changing conditions. The microprocessor is also found in electronic prostheses (replacement limbs and organs). This technology has made possible prosthetic limbs that can receive electrical signals from the residual limb and move. Now fingers can move independently of each other and play the piano; feet can walk and run; hands can feel hot and cold. Computerized functional electrical stimulation (CFES) applied to the outside of a paralyzed limb can simulate a workout and can even return movement to some paralyzed limbs.

Special-Purpose Applications

Computers have made a major, positive contribution to the pharmaceutical industry. Computers can be used in every facet of pharmacy, including helping design medications to warning of possible adverse drug events, filling prescriptions, and delivering medication. They may help in the design of new medications. Rational drug design is based on the assumption that the body is a collection of molecules; when one molecule causes harm, it is necessary to find another molecule to bind to it and correct it. The correcting molecule must fit it like a key to a lock. Numerous calculations can result in a virtual model of the molecule. Before computers, the calculations had to be performed by hand and the model built of wire, which might take years. Now a powerful computer does the calculations in a fraction of the time and simulates the molecule on a computer screen. Computers can also help design drugs by scanning databases of compounds and trying any one drug likely to work—a computer's process of trial and error. Computers made possible the **Human Genome Project**, which sought to understand the genetic makeup of a human being. Part of the Human Genome Project attempted to gain an understanding of the genetic bases of diseases. This understanding could lead to the development of medications.

The use of computers in health-care education is also considered a special-purpose use. Programs such as ADAM and ILIAD have been used for years: ADAM is used to help teach anatomy, and ILIAD teaches clinical-based problem-solving skills. Today simulations are used to help teach skills in dentistry, surgery, and nursing.

There are huge databases of medical information on the Internet. Anyone with an Internet connection can access them. Unfortunately the information on the Internet is not always accurate or credible, and patients must learn to be discerning in the information that they read. That said, due to the amount of knowledge patient's can access on the Internet, the patient may have more up-to-date knowledge of a particular treatment or condition than the doctor. Recommended reputable sites for information include the University of Iowa or the government-maintained MEDLARS databases. The largest of these is MEDLINE, which includes abstracts of articles from around the world and is searchable by using PubMed (MEDLINE's search engine). However reliable the site, individuals should *not* substitute Internet information for a visit to a health-care provider.

Telemedicine

Connectivity and networking have made the field of telemedicine possible. Telemedicine involves the delivery of health care over telecommunications lines. It includes everything from the sharing of radiological images over a network (the oldest form of telemedicine), to distance exams via videoconferencing, to telepsychiatry, teledermatology, teleoncology, and even distance surgery. Via a telemedical hookup, visiting nurses in New Jersey see some patients without leaving the office. A computer named HANC (Home-Assisted Nursing Care) allows a nurse to take blood pressure and listen to a patient's heart without visiting the patient. HANC also reminds the patient to take his or her medicine, speaking louder and louder until the patient responds, and finally, if there is no response, notifying a nurse. Telemedicine delivers health care in some prisons. It is also used in problem pregnancies to get an expert consult without a patient having to wait weeks for an appointment or travel what may be long distances. In addition, telemedicine has been used to deliver psychiatric services to hearing-impaired clients and to deliver health services to a homeless shelter. There have been no comprehensive studies comparing telemedicine and conventional medicine. Early indications are, however, that telemedicine compares favorably with conventional medicine.

Privacy and Security of Medical Information

Computers have made significant contributions to health care and its delivery. But not all of the contributions of computers are positive. Computers and networks endanger the privacy of personal information. Information is kept in databases and on computer networks relative to many aspects of our lives: phone calls we make, property we own, Web sites we visit, our credit card purchases, our marital status, the numbers and ages of our children, our medical records, and our credit status. Much of this information was always gathered. However, it usually was filed away in small courthouses (marriage licenses, property ownership). It was scattered physically and difficult to find. Now much of this information is kept on computer networks, including the Internet. The Medical Information Bureau, an organization made up of insurance companies, keeps the medical records of anyone with insurance. Until April 14, 2003, this information could be shared with other insurance companies and with employers. In April 2003, new regulations regarding the privacy of medical information (discussed later in this chapter) went into effect under the Health Insurance Portability and Accountability Act of 1996 (HIPAA).

The paper medical record is currently being replaced by the **electronic medical record (EMR)**.[*] The EMR may be stored in a hospital's private network, but it may also be kept on the Internet.

There are many benefits to the EMR: your record is available anywhere there is a computer on the network; EMR helps guarantee continuity of care; each of your health-care providers knows your full medical history and can, therefore, provide better care. Let's assume you are in an accident in New Jersey but live in California. Your medical record is a mouse click away. The EMR is legible and complete. However, despite its benefits, the EMR raises serious privacy issues. Any network can be compromised, and your medical information stolen and misused. A great deal of medical information is private. No one wants their psychiatric diagnosis and/or HIV status to become public knowledge. Privacy issues are also raised by telemedicine, which transmits medical information across state lines via telecommunications lines. The states have traditionally provided protection for medical information; however, once the information crosses state lines, it does not have state legal protection.

Are there ways of protecting sensitive information or guaranteeing security? There are various attempts to guarantee that only people authorized to see the information have access. Computers can be kept in a locked room, and authorized personnel can be issued keys or swipe cards; **PINs (personal identification numbers)** and passwords can be used to identify authorized users; **biometric methods** can be used—handprints, fingerprints, face scans, body scans, iris scans; and **encryption** (scrambling) of sensitive data, so only authorized personnel have the **decryption** (unscrambling) software. **Firewalls** (electronic blocks) are used to keep people out of private networks. **Callback systems** are used to attempt to protect networks. A user calls in; the network hangs up and calls the user back at an authorized phone. None of these methods is foolproof. Keys and cards can be lost or stolen; PINs and passwords can be forgotten or shared.

Restricting computer access to people who are authorized is not really enough. The FBI estimates that people who have legitimate access commit more than half of all computer crimes. With our current fragmented health-care system, more and more people are authorized to see a medical record. HMOs (health maintenance organizations) are replacing traditional practice. In one hospital stay, think of how many people share your record—from clerks in a pharmacy, to kitchen personnel in the hospital kitchen, to technicians, nurses, and doctors. Many of these people are not trained in medical ethics and don't fully understand the issues related to protecting a patient's privacy. Of course, it would help to train all hospital personnel in medical ethics, not to share information, and to use password-protected screensavers. However, this would not solve

---

[*]For a complete discussion of medical privacy issues, see Lillian Burke and Barbara Weill, *Information Technology for the Health Professions* (Upper Saddle River, NJ: Prentice Hall, 2009), Chapter 4.

the problem. When a person obtains medical insurance, he or she signs away all privacy rights. Until these privacy and security problems are solved, the EMR will not fulfill its promise to make complete and accurate medical information available to those who need it while fully protecting the patient's privacy.

The Health Insurance Portability and Accountability Act of 1996 (HIPAA)

According to HIPAA's Notice of Privacy Practices for Protected Health Information, **protected health information (PHI)** includes any information that can be used in some manner to identify the person such as a person's Social Security number, ZIP code, and birth date. Under the HIPAA rule, protection of patient health information was established for transaction of claims and remittances, eligibility inquiries and claims status. HIPAA privacy laws require maintaining appropriate administrative, technical, and physical safeguards to ensure the integrity and confidentiality of patient health information. HIPAA security rules identify steps to take to secure PHI that is in electronic format. Equally as important are guidelines to the rights of patients concerning their personal health information. The rules help offices ensure processes are in place to protect the patient information covered by the HIPAA privacy rules.

Federal HIPAA privacy requirements consist of three categories:

1. Privacy standards
2. Patients' rights
3. Administrative requirements

Privacy standards require that as of April 14, 2003, all medical offices must provide a copy of their office's notice of privacy practice to each patient at the first visit to a practice. A copy must also be prominently posted on any Web site the practice maintains. Under HIPAA, the policy states that patients have rights over their own PHI. These rights include the right to the following:

- Access and obtain copies of their PHI
- Amend PHI in their records
- Be notified of nonroutine and nonauthorized disclosure
- Have confidential communications with their care providers
- File complaints to the practice and/or the Secretary of Health and Human Services (HHS).

In the administrative requirement, policies, procedures, and documentation must be created. Every office must have in place a HIPAA privacy contact person who is responsible for providing training in privacy and safeguarding of PHI. Patients may file complaints concerning the PHI with that contact person. Other administrative requirements include the establishment of a complaint system and a system on how to mitigate a complaint if a breach of privacy does occur. When business associates are involved with medical practice agreements, protecting PHI must be contracted and documented within the HIPAA policy manuals.

Compromised PHI penalties handed down from the Health and Human Services Office of Civil Rights can include fines up to $250,000 and ten years' imprisonment. It is important that all medical facilities stay compliant with changes to HIPAA.

Summary

- Computers are used throughout our society, including in health care and its delivery.
- The use of computers in health care and its delivery is called medical informatics.
- Administrative applications include the use of computers in a medical office. MediSoft allows the user to computerize medical office administrative functions.
- Clinical applications use computers in direct patient care such as diagnosis, monitoring, and treatment.
- Special-purpose applications include drug design and educational uses.
- Telemedicine is the delivery of health care over telecommunications lines and includes administrative, clinical, and special-purpose applications.

- Medical information is available online in electronic form. The electronic medical record (EMR) provides continuity of care. The privacy and security issues surrounding the EMR must be addressed. Some attempts at restricting access to medical records include training personnel, PINs and passwords for authorized personnel, encryption, firewalls, and callback systems. Further steps must be taken to guarantee the security of medical information.
- The Health Insurance Portability and Accountability Act (HIPAA) encourages the use of the electronic medical record and provides minimum national standards for the protection of medical information.

Review Exercises

Define the Following Terms:

Medical informatics

Administrative applications

Telemedicine

Clinical applications

Special-purpose applications

Briefly Discuss the Following:

1. Discuss the advantages and disadvantages of the electronic medical record.

2. Discuss the privacy issues associated with telemedicine.

3. HIPAA requires medical offices to design privacy policies. Discuss the safeguards you would introduce to protect the patient's privacy of information.

CHAPTER TWO

A BRIEF INTRODUCTION TO THE WINDOWS ENVIRONMENT

Chapter Outline

- Introduction
- Windows
  - The Parts of a Window
  - The Parts of a Dialog Box
- Summary
- Review Exercises

Learning Objectives

Upon completion of this chapter, the student will:

- Be familiar with the Windows environment and its terminology.
- Be able to describe the parts of a window and a dialog box.

Key Terms

Application software	Hand	Spin Box
Arrow	Hourglass	Status Bar
Booting	I-beam	System Software
Check Boxes	Icon	Tabs
Clicking	List Box	Taskbar
Command Button	Mouse	Text Box
Common User Interface	Option Button	Toolbar
Desktop	Operating System	Two-Headed Arrow
Dialog Box	Pointing	Window
Double-Clicking	Program	Windows
Dragging	Right-Clicking	
Drop-Down List Box	Scroll Bar	
Graphical User Interface (GUI)	Slide Box	
	Software	

Introduction

This chapter introduces basic Windows vocabulary and concepts. MediSoft for Windows operates in a **Windows** environment. It is necessary to be familiar with Windows terminology to fully appreciate and utilize MediSoft.

Windows

Computer hardware cannot function without instructions. These step-by-step instructions are called **programs** or **software**. There are two basic kinds of software: application and system. **Application software** helps to do a specific task; for example, a word-processing program helps you type a letter or memo; MediSoft helps computerize administrative functions in a health-care environment. **System software** takes care of tasks for the computer. The most important piece of system software is the **operating system (OS)**. Every computer has an operating system that takes care of routine tasks and provides a user interface so the user can communicate with the computer's hardware. The operating system coordinates and controls basic input and output, receives commands from the keyboard, and displays information on the screen. It also organizes and tracks your files in memory and on disk. The operating system must be loaded in the computer's memory for the computer to do anything, a process called **booting**.

Today most personal computers use Windows as an operating system. Windows allows the user to communicate with the computer through a **graphical user interface (GUI)** by using a **mouse** and clicking on **icons** (pictures and symbols).

A mouse is an input device attached to the computer by a cable or optically through a receiving device. It has one, two, or three buttons on the top and a ball or optical input on the bottom. When you move the mouse across a flat surface (e.g., a mouse pad), a mouse pointer moves on the screen.

The mouse pointer takes on different shapes:

- An **arrow** ↗ when selecting or choosing

- An **I-beam** I for editing

- An **hourglass** when Windows needs time to process a command

- A **two-headed arrow** ↔ when changing the size of a window

- A **hand** to choose help topics

There are several basic mouse operations:

- **Pointing** is moving the mouse to point at a particular item.

- **Clicking** is pressing and releasing the left mouse button.

- **Double-clicking** is quickly pressing and releasing the left mouse button twice.

- **Right-clicking** is clicking the right mouse button. It often opens a shortcut menu.

- **Dragging** is holding down the left mouse button while moving the mouse.

Your work area, the screen on which icons and windows are arranged, is called the **desktop**. Across the bottom of the desktop is a **taskbar**. The taskbar displays a button for each open application. At the left of the taskbar is a Start button. Clicking Start causes a menu (list of choices) to pop up. You can execute most tasks by sliding the mouse pointer to the option you want and clicking. If an option has a right-pointing arrowhead next to it, another menu will drop down; move the mouse pointer to that menu, slide it to your selection, and click.

When you first launch Windows, there are several icons on the desktop. An icon is a little picture representing a program or piece of hardware. To open an icon into a window (a rectangular area surrounded by a border), point to the icon and double-click. In Windows, applications (programs) run in Windows and Documents open in Windows.

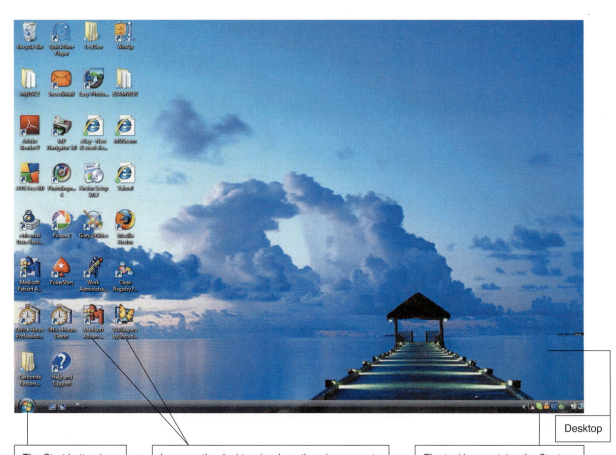

Desktop

The Start button is the first thing on the taskbar. It allows the user to access programs and shut down the computer.

Icons on the desktop (such as these) represent program or hardware. Icons can be opened into windows by pointing and double-clicking.

The taskbar contains the Start button, and a button for every running application. On this taskbar, you can see buttons for WordPerfect, Windows, and Paint.

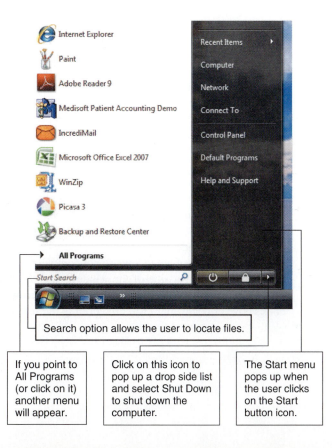

Search option allows the user to locate files.

If you point to All Programs (or click on it) another menu will appear.

Click on this icon to pop up a drop side list and select Shut Down to shut down the computer.

The Start menu pops up when the user clicks on the Start button icon.

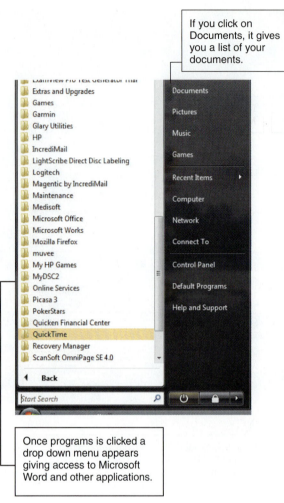

If you click on Documents, it gives you a list of your documents.

Once programs is clicked a drop down menu appears giving access to Microsoft Word and other applications.

The Parts of a Window

One of the features of the Windows environment is a **common user interface**; this means that every window has similar parts. Across the top is a title bar with the window title in it. At the right of the title bar are three buttons: the minimize, maximize or restore, and close buttons. Clicking the minimize button does not cause the application to stop running; the button still appears on the taskbar, although you no longer see an open window. The maximize button causes the window to expand to fill the screen. When a window is maximized, a restore button to replace the maximize button is provided. Clicking the restore button causes the window to resume its former size. Clicking the close button closes the window; the application is no longer running, and its button is no longer on the taskbar.

Some windows have other components. Below the title bar (in windows that run applications) is a menu bar. **Toolbars** may appear below the menu bar and let you execute a command by clicking on a button. Across the bottom of some windows, a **status bar** gives you information about the open window.

If the contents of a window are not completely visible, **scroll bars** appear across the bottom and/or down the right side of the window. A scroll bar contains two scroll arrows and a scroll box. To move through a window, click on the arrow pointing in the direction you want to go, click above or below the scroll box, or drag the scroll box.

The Parts of a Window

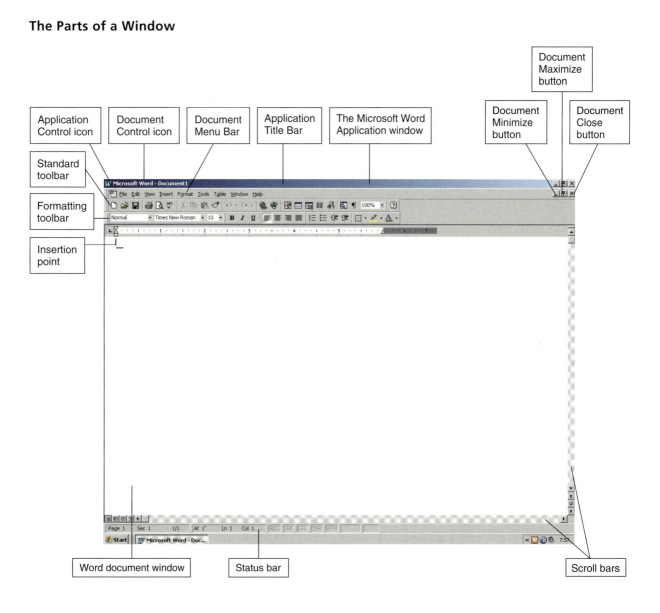

A menu is a list of commands. You can choose an item from the menu by highlighting it and pressing the Enter key or by simply pointing to the item with the mouse and clicking the left mouse button. When you choose a command that is followed by an ellipsis (three dots . . .), the command is not immediately executed. Instead, a window called a **dialog box** opens. A dialog box is a window used when the computer needs more information. Dialog boxes may have one or more of the following elements:

- **Tabs** look like file folder tabs. They appear at the top of the dialog box and are used to switch to a different page of the dialog box.
- **Text boxes** allow you to enter data.
- **List boxes** display a list of choices. Click on the option to make a choice.
- **Drop-down list boxes** contain a down arrow; click on the arrow to display the choices. Click on the option to make a choice.
- **Command buttons** are rectangular buttons that execute commands. OK and Cancel are common.
- **Check boxes** are square boxes that you can click on or off. More than one may be chosen.
- **Option buttons** are round. Only one may be selected; however, one *must* be selected.
- **Spin boxes** allow you to make a choice by clicking on an up or down arrow.
- **Slide boxes** let you to make a choice by moving a slider bar.

The Parts of a Dialog Box

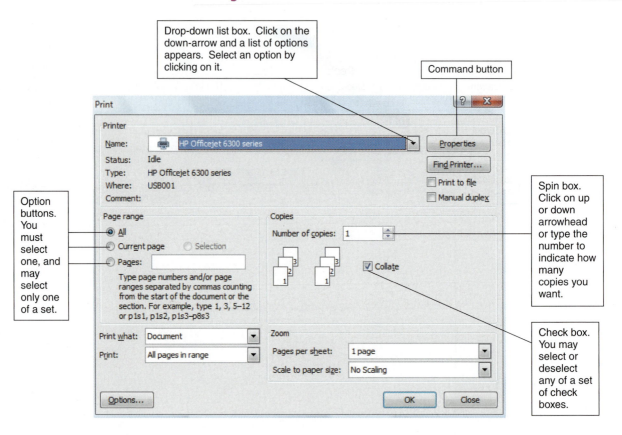

Drop-down list box. Click on the down-arrow and a list of options appears. Select an option by clicking on it.

Command button

Option buttons. You must select one, and may select only one of a set.

Spin box. Click on up or down arrowhead or type the number to indicate how many copies you want.

Check box. You may select or deselect any of a set of check boxes.

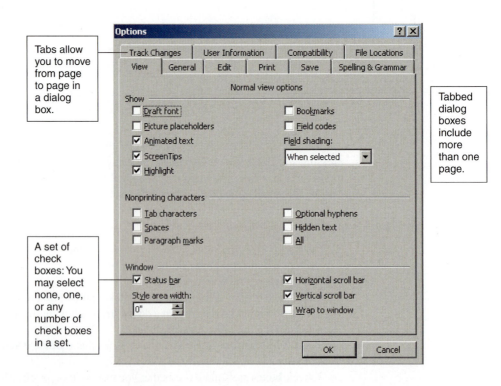

Tabs allow you to move from page to page in a dialog box.

Tabbed dialog boxes include more than one page.

A set of check boxes: You may select none, one, or any number of check boxes in a set.

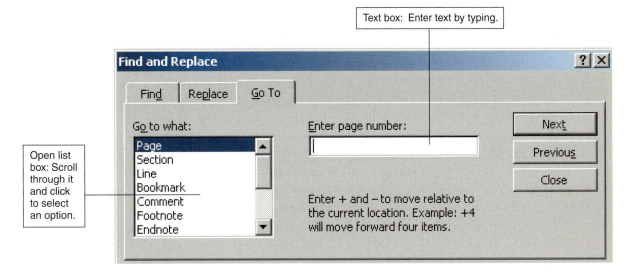

Text box: Enter text by typing.

Open list box: Scroll through it and click to select an option.

Summary

- The operating system is a piece of system software that defines the general working environment of a computer. Therefore, it is necessary for the user to be familiar with the operating system. Application software helps you do a specific task. MediSoft is an application program that helps computerize functions in a medical office environment. The following chapters will introduce the user to MediSoft in a Windows environment.

Review Exercises

Fill-in Questions

1. A window called a _____ is used to collect more information for the computer.
2. The user must make _____ choice(s) from a group of option buttons.
3. _____ appear across the top of a many-paged dialog box.
4. A user may choose many or none from a group of _____ boxes.
5. Windows provides a _____ user interface. The user controls a mouse to click on icons.

True/False Questions

1. Windows is an example of system software called an operating system. T/F
2. Booting refers to loading any program into memory. T/F

3. The user is required to make one choice from a set of option buttons. T/F
4. The user must make one choice from a set of four check boxes. T/F

Matching Questions

Match the letter from the illustration below with the correct name:

_____ Formatting toolbar   _____ Title bar

_____ Application control icon   _____ Minimize button

_____ Menu bar   _____ Standard toolbar

_____ Close button   _____ Maximize button

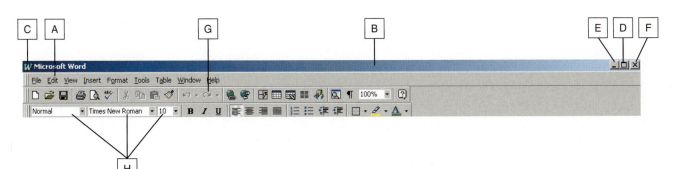

CHAPTER THREE

AN OVERVIEW: USING MEDISOFT IN THE MEDICAL OFFICE

Chapter Outline

- Introduction
- Database Concepts
- An Overview of MediSoft
  - The Patient Information Form
  - Coding Systems: ICD, CPT, and DRG
  - The Electronic Medical Record
  - Accounting, Using MediSoft
  - Insurance
  - Claims
  - Accounting Reports
- Summary
- Review Exercises

Learning Objectives

Upon completion of this chapter, the student will be able to:

- Define basic database terms, including *file, table, record,* and *field*.
- Understand the flow of work in a medical office from the patient information form to the electronic medical record to the submission of insurance claims.
- Define the coding systems (DRG, ICD, CPT) and understand their uses.
- Describe the role of MediSoft in the accounting process.
- Comprehend the differences between types of insurance (fee-for-service, health maintenance organizations, capitated plans, participating provider organizations, etc.).
- Understand the process of claims submission.
- Explain MediSoft's various accounting reports.

Key Terms

Accounts Receivable (A/R)	Bucket Billing	CHAMPVA
Adjustment	Capitated Plan	Charge
Assignment	Case	Claim
Authorization	Center for Medicare and Medicaid Services (CMS)	Clearinghouse
Balance Billing		CMS-1500

Copayment

CPT (Current Procedural Terminology)

Database

Database Management Software (DBMS)

Deductible

Diagnosis-Related Group (DRG)

Electronic Medical Record (EMR)

Electronic Remittance Advice (ERA)

Electronic Media Claim (EMC)

Encounter Form

Explanation of Benefits (EOB)

Fee-for-Service Plan

Field

File

Guarantor

Health Maintenance Organization (HMO)

ICD-9-CM (International Classification of Diseases, 9th Edition, Clinical Modifications)

Indemnity Plan

Key Field

Managed Care

Medicaid

Medicare

Patient Aging Applied Payment

Patient Aging Report

Patient Day Sheet

Payment

Payment Day Sheet

Practice Analysis Report

Preferred Provider Organization (PPO)

Procedure Day Sheet

Record

Schedule of Benefits

Superbill

Table

Transaction

TRICARE

Worker's Compensation

X12 837

Introduction

MediSoft can be used by medical administrators, office workers, doctors, other health care workers, and students. It can greatly ease the tasks of administering a practice using a computer. The amount of data and information a modern practice has to collect and organize is overwhelming. MediSoft allows the user to computerize tasks performed every day in any medical environment. All the disparate tasks and pieces of data and information need to be well organized, accessible, and easily linked. Because MediSoft is a relational database, the user can quickly and easily organize, access, and link information used in the various parts of the program.

Database Concepts

A **database** is an organized collection of information. **Database management software (DBMS)** allows the user to enter, organize, and store huge amounts of data and information. The information can then be updated, sorted, and retrieved. In order to use DBMS efficiently, the user should be familiar with certain concepts and definitions. A database **file** holds all related information on an entity, for example, a medical practice. Within each file, there can be several **tables**. Each table holds related information; for example, one table might hold information on a practice's doctors; another, information on its patients; another, information on its insurance carriers. A table is made up of related **records**; each record holds all the information on one item in a table. For example, each patient has a record in the practice's patient table, and all the information on that patient makes up that patient's record. Each record is comprised up of related **fields**. Each field holds a single piece of information, such as a patient's last name, Social Security number (SSN), or chart number. One field—the **key field**—uniquely identifies each record in a table. The information in that field cannot be duplicated. The Social Security number is a common key field because no two people have the same SSN. The chart number uniquely identifies each patient's chart. In a relational database such as MediSoft, related tables are linked by sharing a common field.

An Overview of MediSoft

MediSoft allows the user to create one database file for each practice. Within each database, information is organized in tables. The tables are linked by sharing a common field.

The Patient Information Form

When a patient schedules an appointment, it is recorded in MediSoft's Electronic Appointment Book. At or before a patient's first visit, he fills out a Patient Information Form. It includes personal data such as name, address, contact phone numbers, date of birth, and Social Security number. The patient is also asked to fill in information about his spouse or partner.

In addition, the patient is asked to provide insurance information for himself and a spouse or partner. This information includes the name of the primary, secondary, and tertiary insurance carriers, name and birth date of the policyholder, the copayment, and policy and group numbers.

Coding Systems: ICD, CPT, and DRG

Categories of information on patients such as personal, medical, and insurance information when entered into MediSoft become part of the patient record. Some of it is translated into codes before it is entered. Codes provide standardization that allows the easy sharing of information. Codes for diagnoses and procedures are precise and universally used, allowing physicians to communicate clearly regarding the types of procedures performed and patient diagnoses.

Services including office visits, tests, lab work, exams, and treatments are coded using the most up-to-date **current procedural terminology (CPT)** codes. The **ICD-9-CM** (*International Classification of Diseases*, ninth edition, *Clinical Modification*) provides three-, four-, or five-digit codes for more than a thousand diseases. Both the CPT and ICD-9-CM coding systems make electronic claims forms easier to file because each condition or disease, service, procedure, and diagnostic test can readily be identified by established codes. There is no reason for every practice to use every code in its database. When a new practice is set up, only codes that relate to its specialty are entered in one of the tables of codes; these tables can always be amended. The CPT codes that are most frequently used by the medical office are preprinted on the encounter form (also called the superbill). Some practices also print the diagnosis codes on this form.

Standard coding systems include **diagnosis-related group (DRG)**. Today hospital reimbursement by private and government insurers is determined by diagnosis. Each patient is given a DRG classification and a formula based on this classification that determines reimbursement. If hospital care and cost exceed the prospective cost determination, the hospital absorbs the financial loss.

The Electronic Medical Record

The information that was gathered from the patient is entered into the computer and forms the patient's medical record. The electronic medical record (EMR) is starting to replace the paper record. Hospital owned medical offices are currently in the process of switching from the hardcopy patient medical record to the EMR. Hospital owned medical offices are in the process currently of switching from the hard copy patient medical record to the EMR.

Accounting, Using MediSoft

MediSoft is essentially an accounting program. Therefore, several definitions are required. **Charges**, **payments**, and **adjustments** are called **transactions**. A charge is simply the amount a patient is billed for the provider's service. A payment is made by a patient or an insurance carrier to the practice. An adjustment is a positive or negative change to a patient's account. Transactions are organized around cases. A **case** is the condition for which the patient visits the doctor. There can be several visits associated with one case. There can also be several cases (one for each diagnosis) for one patient. The medical office staff enters information for a patient's case in MediSoft where it is stored in the practice's database tables. When you add a case, the patient's insurance information is entered. Due to this fact, it is important to create a new case if the patient's insurance changes. A case can be closed when the patient's condition is resolved.

Insurance

Today many people are covered by medical insurance. Those people who are not covered either pay out of pocket or seek care in the local emergency room. A **guarantor** is the person responsible for payment; it may be the patient or a third party. There is a variety of options for those with insurance.

INDEMNITY AND FEE-FOR-SERVICE PLANS Some carriers have a **schedule of benefits**—a list of those services that the carrier will cover—called an **indemnity plan**. Indemnity plans are becoming less common because they are **fee-for-service plans** and, therefore, are very expensive. The patient is never restricted to a network of providers and needs no referrals for specialists. In an indemnity plan, the patient must fulfill a **deductible** (a certain amount the patient is required to pay each year before the insurance carrier begins paying). The patient is also responsible for her portion of the coinsurance, which is the amount of the allowable charge once the insurance carrier pays its percentage of the bill and determines the allowable charge.

MANAGED CARE ORGANIZATIONS Managed care plans are fixed, prepaid plans with contracted health care providers obtained either independently or as a group. **Managed care** has a schedule of benefits for out-of-network providers. There are several forms of managed care. Managed care organizations include health maintenance organizations (HMOs) and preferred provider organizations (PPOs).

A patient who uses an HMO pays a fixed yearly fee and must choose from an approved network of health care providers and hospitals. The patient must designate a primary care provider (PCP), who must make a referral before the patient can see a specialist. If a patient goes out of network without the HMO's approval, the patient must pay all costs out of pocket.

PPOs may require that the provider get **authorization** before a procedure is performed. This is simply permission by the insurance carrier for the provider to perform a medical procedure. A patient with PPO insurance can seek care within an approved network of health care providers who have agreed with the insurance company to lower their charges and accept **assignment** (the contracted dollar amount the insurance company pays). The patient pays a small fee called a **copayment**, the part of the charge for which the patient is responsible. The patient may choose to go out of network but will receive reduced reimbursement.

In a **capitated plan**, a physician is paid a fixed fee (the capitation). The capitation is based on the number of patients assigned to the physician in a given month. The provider is then paid a flat fee whether or not all patients are seen. Some patients may seek no treatment; some may visit several times.

MEDICAID There are several government insurance plans. They are administered by the federal **Center for Medicare and Medicaid Services** (**CMS**, www.cms.hhs.gov). Each year millions of Americans receive health care through government insurers—some through fee-for-service plans, some through managed care. According to the U.S. Department of Health and Human Resources, **Medicaid** is "an assistance program. Medical bills are paid from federal, state and local tax funds. It serves low-income people of every age. Patients usually pay no part of costs for covered medical expenses. A small co-payment is sometimes required" (www.hhs.gov/faq/medicaremedicaid). Medicaid resembles managed care in that the patient is restricted to a network of providers, must get a authorization for procedures, and needs referrals to any specialist.

MEDICARE Medicare coverage is dependent not on one's income level, but rather on one's age. **Medicare** mostly serves people age sixty-five and older and disabled people with chronic renal disorders. Medicare allows patients to choose their physicians; referrals are not needed. Many people supplement Medicare with private fee-for-service plans in which they are not restricted to a network of providers and do not need referrals to specialists. The patient is required to pay a copay, and the provider bills the insurance for the remainder. Some Medicare patients choose to belong to a Medicare HMO.

OTHER GOVERNMENT PROGRAMS **CHAMPVA** and **TRICARE** are federal health benefits programs that supplement medical care for military personnel and/or dependants and widows. **Worker's compensation** is a government program that covers job-related illness or injury.

Claims

To receive payment for services from an uninsured patient, the practice simply bills the patient. To receive payment for services rendered to an insured patient, the practice must submit a **claim** to the insurance carrier. A claim is a request to an insurance company for payment for services. If an insurance carrier requires a treatment plan, the current version of MediSoft enables you to create one. The hardcopy insurance claim form is called the **CMS-1500**. An **electronic media claim (EMC)** is an electronically processed and transmitted claim and is called an X12 837.

To create a claim, the practice needs to gather certain information: the patient's condition, the physician's diagnosis, and the procedures performed in the office or hospital. The patient record provides personal data, medical history, and insurance information. The provider table can supply information about the physician. Claims are submitted on paper or electronically. Practices that submit electronic claims use a **clearinghouse**—a business that collects insurance claims from providers and sends them to the correct insurance carrier. An insurance company can reject the claim or send a check for partial or full payment. The response to a claim includes an **explanation of benefits (EOB)** to the patient and an electronic remittance advice (ERA) that explains why certain services were covered and others not. The practice records the claim remittance and applies it to the charge. Then it bills the secondary insurer; the EOB from the first insurer is sent to the secondary insurer with the claim. (Most of this happens via electronic submission and is handled automatically by the software.) The secondary insurer responds with a check and EOB or ERA. After the response is received from the secondary insurer, the tertiary insurance company is billed. It is only after the response is received from all of a patient's carriers that the patient is billed. This is called bucket billing or balance billing. MediSoft is structured to handle bucket billing, which is unique to the health-care environment.

From the time a patient is charged for a procedure to the time when all payments have been received and credited to the patient's account, there is a sequence of accounting events that occur. **Accounts receivable (A/R)** include any invoices outstanding or any payments from the patient or insurance carriers to the medical practice. The diagnoses and procedures relevant to a patient's visit are recorded on an **encounter form** (also called a **superbill**). Encounter forms are printed for the scheduled appointments either the night before or the morning of and their data is used in several MediSoft accounting reports.

Accounting Reports

MediSoft provides the user with various kinds of reports that are generated on a daily, monthly, or yearly basis. Daily reports include a **patient day sheet**, a **procedure day sheet**, and a **payment day sheet**. A patient day sheet lists the day's patients, chart numbers, and transactions. It is used for daily reconciliation. A procedure day sheet is a report organized by procedure. Patients who underwent a particular procedure are listed under that procedure. This report is used to see what procedures each provider is performing. It also can be used to find the most profitable procedures. A payment day sheet is a grouped report organized by providers. Each patient is listed under his provider. It shows the amounts received from each patient to each provider.

A **practice analysis report**, generated on a monthly basis, is a management tool for tracking procedures performed, payments received, and adjustments made to accounts for those procedures during a specified period (MediSoft Help Tool).

MediSoft provides two patient aging reports: **Patient Aging** and **Patient Aging Applied Payment**. These two similar reports help identify accounts with balances that are past due. The former includes unapplied payments in the totals but has no Date from Range filter, and the latter excludes unapplied payments and has a Date from Range filter (MediSoft Help Tool).

The administrative and accounting tasks of a health-care environment can be computerized using MediSoft. It allows the user to enter all necessary information into tables, link the information, and present it in one of the many reports it provides. Computerizing the accounting transactions allows the office to avoid being buried in paper and keeps all accounts in an accurate, up-to-date, and well-organized structure.

Summary

- The flow of work in a medical office may start with a call from someone wanting to make an appointment. It can be recorded in MediSoft's electronic appointment book. The patient fills out a patient information form, and this information is then entered into a computer. Once the patient is seen and diagnosed, that information is also recorded electronically.
- The information collected on the patient information form includes name, address, phone number, Social Security number, insurance information, relationship to the insured, working information, and so on.
- Coding systems include the CPT, ICD-9-CM, and DRG.
- The paper record is being replaced by the electronic medical record (EMR).
- Accounting functions in a medical office include bucket (balance) billing; sending claims; and recording charges, payments, and deposits. MediSoft can help streamline and structure these functions.

- There are several types of medical insurance, including Medicare, Medicaid, fee-for-service, and managed care organizations.
- Most claims are filed electronically (form X12 837), but claims can also be filed as a hardcopy (form CMS-1500).
- MediSoft makes it easy to generate several kinds of accounting reports, such as the patient day sheet, procedure day sheet, payment day sheet, practice analysis, and patient aging reports.

Review Exercises

Matching Exercises

Match the term with its definition.

1. Electronic media claim (EMC) _____
2. Explanation of benefits (EOB) _____
3. Center for Medicare and Medicaid Services (CMS) _____
4. Clearinghouse _____
5. Superbill _____
6. Practice analysis report _____
7. Patient aging report _____
8. Authorization _____
9. Managed care _____
10. DRG _____
11. CPT _____
12. ICD-9-CM _____
13. CMS-1500 _____
14. Patient day sheet _____
15. Schedule of benefits _____

A. Form returned by an insurance carrier that explains why certain services were covered and others were not.
B. Insurance plan in which insurance carrier determines what treatment is necessary and pays for it.
C. Formula based on this code helps determine reimbursement.
D. List of those services that the carrier will cover.
E. Coding system for services including tests, lab work, exams, and treatments.
F. The most widely accepted insurance form.
G. Federal agency that administers Medicaid and Medicare.
H. Report used to show a patient's outstanding payments.
I. Form on which diagnoses and procedures relevant to a patient's visit are recorded (also called an encounter form).
J. Report generated on a monthly basis; it is a summary total of all procedures, charges, and transactions.
K. Business that collects insurance claims from providers and sends them to the correct insurance carrier.
L. Electronically processed and transmitted claim.
M. Three-, four-, or five-digit codes for more than a thousand diseases.
N. Permission by the insurance carrier for the provider to perform a medical procedure, that is, the insurance company deems it necessary and will cover it.
O. Report that lists the day's patients, chart numbers, and transactions.

Define the Following Terms:

1. Field
2. Record
3. Table
4. Database
5. Key Field

CHAPTER FOUR

A HANDS-ON INTRODUCTION TO MEDISOFT AND THE APPOINTMENT BOOK

Chapter Outline

- The MediSoft Window
- Getting Started
  - Making an Appointment: Office Hours
  - The Office Hours Toolbar
  - A Note About Dates
  - The Office Hours Window
  - Making an Appointment
  - Break Entry
  - Entering Repeating Appointments
  - Finding the Next Available Time
  - Printing Appointments
  - The Patient Recall List
- Summary
- Review Exercises

Learning Objectives

Upon completion of this chapter, the student will:

- Be familiar with the MediSoft window and toolbar.
- Be familiar with the office hours window and toolbar.
- Know how to change the MediSoft date.
- Know how to use MediSoft's office hours program.
- Be able to enter appointments, breaks, and repeating appointments.
- Be able to print an appointment schedule.
- Be able to create a patient recall list.

Key Terms

Appointment Grid	MediSoft Date	Sidebar
Appointment List	Office Hours	Windows System Date
Electronic Appointment Book	Patient Recall List	
Global Command	Repeating Appointment	

The MediSoft Window

To launch MediSoft, do the following:

- Double-click the MediSoft icon on the Windows desktop.

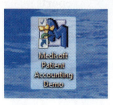

You will see the MediSoft window with the MediSoft title and the words *Tutorial Data* within the title bar:

Title Bar   Menu Bar   Tool Bar

Medisoft Demo - Medical Group (Tutorial Data)

File Edit Activities Lists Reports Tools Window Services Help

F1 Help

July 11, 2008

Function Help Line   Status Bar

Below the title bar, the menu bar contains the names of the pull-down menus. You pull down a menu by clicking on its name.

- The **file menu** contains many options. The most commonly used options are the following:
  - Open practice opens the database for an established practice.
  - New practice sets up a new database for a new practice.
  - Other options allow the user to back up and restore data, set the program date, enter practice information, and perform file management tasks.
- The **edit menu** (which is enabled once information is placed within a field) contains options to cut, copy, paste, and delete information.

- The **activities menu** contains options that allow the user to manage finances, insurance claims, and appointments, and to enter patient, diagnosis, procedure, and case information.
- The **lists menu** contains options that allow the user to enter and edit patient, case, and procedure/payment information; adjustment codes; diagnosis; insurance and billing codes; and information on providers and referring providers.
- The **reports menu** contains a list of predefined reports as well as custom reports and bills that the user can design. Almost all printing is done from the reports menu.
- The **tools menu** gives the user access to a calculator and the contents of a file. The tools menu also allows the user to create reports, customize menu bars, and view system information.
- The **window menu** resembles the window menu in any Windows application, allowing the user to switch between open windows (see Chapter 2).
- The **services menu** provides information on subscribing to and retrieving updates for the prescription-writing service OnCallData™ NDC Health.
- The user can find assistance from the MediSoft **help menu**.

Beneath the menu bar is the **MediSoft toolbar** (sometimes called the **speed bar**). The toolbar icons function in MediSoft in the same way that they function in any Windows application; they give the user fast access to common functions.

The MediSoft Toolbar

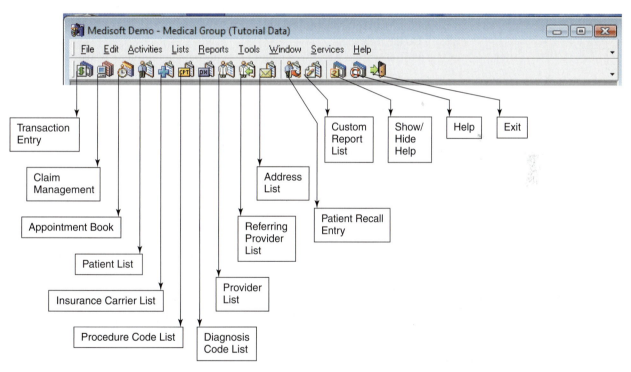

The taskbar is at the bottom of the Windows desktop and contains the Start button, a clock, and buttons for each open application.

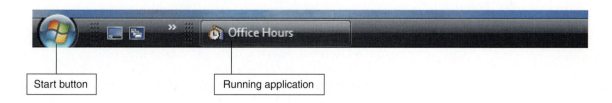

Immediately above the taskbar is the status bar, which provides context-specific information, such as the page number and the date.

Above the status bar is the function help line (also called the shortcut bar), which contains commonly used function keys. In MediSoft, function keys work as **global commands**— commands that work from any point in the program:

- F1   Opens Help files in most windows
- F3   Save
- F6   Opens a search window
- F7   Opens the Quick Ledger window
- F8   Opens a window to create a new record
- F9   Opens a window to edit the selected record
- F11   Opens the Quick Balance window
- ESC   Closes or cancels current function or window

Function key shortcuts are accessed via the keyboard rather than clicking on an icon with the mouse.

Getting Started

Making an Appointment: Office Hours

If you are not looking at the MediSoft window, launch MediSoft by double-clicking on its icon on the desktop. The first contact between the prospective patient and a health-care provider's office is the phone call to set up an appointment. The medical office worker who responds needs to access MediSoft's **electronic appointment book**.

Do the following:

Pull down the Activities menu and choose Appointment Book, or simply click on the

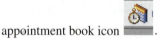

appointment book icon   .

The **office hours** program and MediSoft's two-paned appointment scheduling module window will appear.

Make sure the window title reads *Office Hours—Medical Group (Tutorial Data)*. At the beginning we will be working with tutorial data provided by MediSoft.

The Office Hours Toolbar

Once you have the office hours window on your screen, you will see that a toolbar is provided. As in the MediSoft program, the office hours software allows you quick access into various areas by selecting the appropriate icon.

Office Hours Toolbar

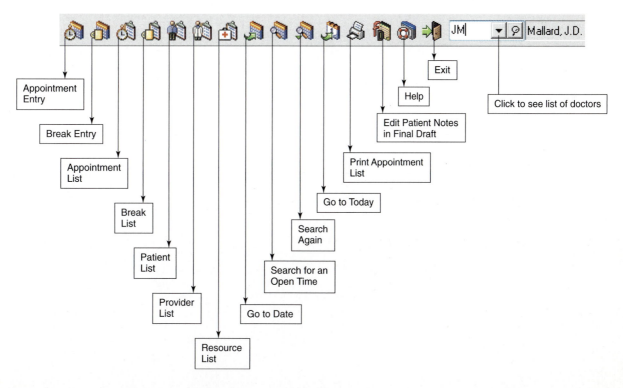

A Note About Dates

MediSoft works with two dates: the **Windows system date** (today's date) on the taskbar, and the **MediSoft date** (the date the health-care administrator is using) on the status bar. Because in some health-care environments not all transactions are entered on the date they occurred, you need to know how to set the MediSoft date so it is correct for the data for which you are entering information.

To change the MediSoft date: Double-click the date on the status bar, and a calendar will pop up. Change the month using the left or right arrow and change the day by clicking on the day you want. Press Enter. The year can be changed by clicking on the year shown.

You should not change the Windows system date. That can cause unforeseen errors in your software.

The Office Hours Window

Office Hours is MediSoft's appointment scheduling software and comes in basic and professional versions. The professional version has added options and is sold separately from MediSoft. Office Hours can be launched by double-clicking on its icon on the Windows desktop or within MediSoft. It can also be launched by clicking on Appointment Book in the Activities menu or the Appointment Book icon, which has a clock face.

Office Hours displays one month's calendar with today's date highlighted in the left pane.

The right pane displays several columns for the appointments. The columns are not for multiple bookings; they are meant for a health-care practice with several providers. You can

move the calendar backward and forward using the arrow keys. Notice that on the appointment side, blocks of time are set aside and color coded for activities that happen each day (e.g., lunch), for appointments with patients, and for other events. The appointment book toolbar contains icons that give quick access to common functions.

In Office Hours Professional, icons at the bottom of the window allow the user to change the view of the calendar.

The default choice, displayed on the Office Hours window, is the current month's calendar on the left and the day's appointment calendar on the right.

When the second icon from the left is clicked, a one month's calendar on the left is displayed and displayed on the right is a week's appointment schedule with appointments and other events indicated for the provider listed on the toolbar.

The next icon when clicked displays the month's calendar on the left; on the right every day of the month appears.

In an office where multiple providers have appointments scheduled, the last icon offers the capability of viewing appointment schedules for all the providers for the day selected.

To return to a view of one day, click on the icon furthest to the right .

Click the down-arrow to select a provider. The following will appear:

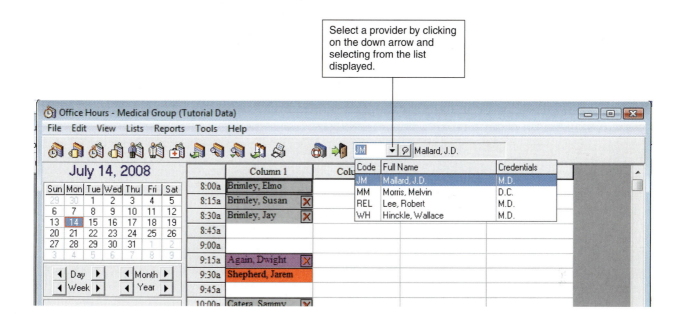

Select a provider by clicking on the down arrow and selecting from the list displayed.

Making an Appointment

Using MediSoft Office Hours, select a provider from the drop-down provider list box. Double-click on 8:30 AM. The New Appointment Entry dialog box will appear.

Fill in the information requested either by using drop-down lists (for the chart number, resource) or by entering information. After selecting the patient, press tab, and MediSoft should automatically fill in the phone number, date, time, case number with corresponding description, length, and provider. Fill in the reason for the appointment by clicking on the reason drop-down list and selecting existing patient for the description. Save the appointment.

As soon as you save the appointment, it appears on the day's appointment calendar.

Break Entry

To enter a break, for example, a lunch break that occurs every day, click on the time (12:00 PM) then click on the Break Entry icon. In the break list window, click on New. The following dialog box will appear. Fill in lunch and make sure All Columns and All Providers are checked. Click on the Change box and indicate that lunch takes place weekly, Monday–Friday. Prior to exiting the Change dialog box, click OK.

Click Save and the following will appear:

Entering Repeating Appointments

To enter **repeating appointments**, the user can click on the Go to Date icon 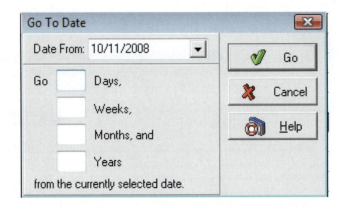 on the appointment book toolbar.

You can instruct the program to display a date that is any number of days, weeks, months, or years from today's date to make an appointment that needs to be periodically repeated. For example, if you go to a date seven days from now, that day's appointment calendar will be displayed and you can enter the appointment.

NOTE: WHEN A DATE NEEDS TO BE ENTERED IN THE GO TO DATE DIALOG BOX, ENTER IT IN AN EIGHT-DIGIT FORMAT: MMDDYYYY. YOU MUST USE THE FOUR DIGITS OF THE YEAR (E.G., 2008).

Dwight Again, as he is leaving on October 11, asks for an appointment in a week. Click on the Go to Date icon and fill in 7 in go _____ days, then click Go. This will bring the calendar for October 18 onto the screen, and you can enter an appointment.

Finding the Next Available Time

If you need to find the next open appointment, you can click Find Open Time in the Office Hours Edit menu, or you can click the Search for Open Time Slot icon on the toolbar. (Hovering over an icon causes a description to appear in the bottom left corner of the window.) Click on the icon now. A dialog box will be displayed.

The patient needs an 8:45 AM appointment on Friday. Click on the day (Friday), fill in the start time (8:45 AM), and click Search. The next available open time slot on a Friday at 8:45 AM will be surrounded by a heavy border. Double-click the time slot, and this dialog box appears:

You need to fill in the chart number by typing in the first few letters of the patient's last name. If a second appointment is needed, click on the Search Again icon. Each time you use Search Again, it brings you to the next available time slot on a Friday at 8:45 AM.

Printing Appointments

To print the day's appointment list, click on the Printer icon then click OK.

In MediSoft Office Hours Professional, you can easily print the **appointment grid** for the day or the week. To print the week's grid, make sure you are looking at the week's calendar. This is done by clicking on View on the menu bar and then Week View. Once you are viewing the entire week of appointments, click on Reports on the menu bar and select Print Appointment Grid. From the fly-out menu, choose Print in Grid View. The following will print:

Appointments

Happy Valley Medical Clinic   Mallard, J.D.   September 7, 2008 - September 13, 2008

	Sunday 7th	Monday 8th	Tuesday 9th	Wednesday 10th	Thursday 11th	Friday 12th	Saturday 13th
8:00a		Brimley, Elmo	Brimley, Elmo	Brimley, Elmo	Brimley, Elmo	Brimley, Elmo	
8:15a		Brimley, Susan	Brimley, Susan	Brimley, Susan	Brimley, Susan	Brimley, Susan	
8:30a		Brimley, Jay	Brimley, Jay	Brimley, Jay	Brimley, Jay	Brimley, Jay	
8:45a							
9:00a							
9:15a		Again, Dwight	Again, Dwight	Again, Dwight	Again, Dwight	Again, Dwight	
9:30a		Shepherd, Jarem	Shepherd, Jarem	Shepherd, Jarem	Shepherd, Jarem	Shepherd, Jarem	
9:45a							
10:00a		Catera, Sammy	Catera, Sammy	Catera, Sammy	Catera, Sammy	Catera, Sammy	
10:15a		Austin, Andrew	Austin, Andrew	Austin, Andrew	Austin, Andrew	Austin, Andrew	
10:30a		Doe, Jane S	Doe, Jane S	Doe, Jane S	Doe, Jane S	Doe, Jane S	
10:45a		Jones, Suzy Q	Jones, Suzy Q	Jones, Suzy Q	Jones, Suzy Q	Jones, Suzy Q	
11:00a		Lunch	Lunch	Lunch	Lunch	Lunch	
11:15a							
11:30a							
11:45a							
12:00p							
12:15p							
12:30p							
12:45p							
1:00p		Peters, Anthony	Peters, Anthony	Peters, Anthony	Peters, Anthony	Peters, Anthony	
1:15p		Peters, Monica C	Peters, Monica C	Peters, Monica C	Peters, Monica C	Peters, Monica C	
1:30p		Peters, Zach	Peters, Zach	Peters, Zach	Peters, Zach	Peters, Zach	
1:45p							
2:00p		Bordon, John	Bordon, John	Bordon, John	Bordon, John	Bordon, John	
2:15p		Gooding, Charles	Gooding, Charles	Gooding, Charles	Gooding, Charles	Gooding, Charles	
2:30p		Simpson, Tanus J	Simpson, Tanus J	Simpson, Tanus J	Simpson, Tanus J	Simpson, Tanus J	
2:45p		Clinger, Wallace	Clinger, Wallace	Clinger, Wallace	Clinger, Wallace	Clinger, Wallace	
3:00p		Jasper, Stephani	Jasper, Stephani	Jasper, Stephani	Jasper, Stephani	Jasper, Stephani	
3:15p		Jacks, Theodore	Jacks, Theodore	Jacks, Theodore	Jacks, Theodore	Jacks, Theodore	
3:30p							
3:45p							
4:00p		Karvel, Jessica C	Karvel, Jessica C	Karvel, Jessica C	Karvel, Jessica C	Karvel, Jessica C	
4:15p		Doogan, James	Doogan, James	Doogan, James	Doogan, James	Doogan, James	
4:30p		Zimmerman, Anth	Zimmerman, Anth	Zimmerman, Anth	Zimmerman, Anth	Zimmerman, Anth	
4:45p		Palmdale, Timoth	Palmdale, Timoth	Palmdale, Timoth	Palmdale, Timoth	Palmdale, Timoth	

Printed 7/14/2008 1:13 pm

To print the day's appointment grid, make sure you are looking at the day's calendar by selecting Day View from the View menu bar. Pull down the Reports menu and choose Print Appointment Grid. The following will print:

Appointments

Happy Valley Medical Clinic   Mallard, J.D.   September 12, 2008

	Column 1	Column 2	Column 3
8:00a	Brimley, Elmo		
8:15a	Brimley, Susan		
8:30a	Brimley, Jay		
8:45a			
9:00a			
9:15a	Again, Dwight		
9:30a	Shepherd, Jarem		
9:45a			
10:00a	Catera, Sammy		
10:15a	Austin, Andrew		
10:30a	Doe, Jane S		
10:45a	Jones, Suzy Q		
11:00a	Lunch	Lunch	Lunch
11:15a			
11:30a			
11:45a			
12:00p			
12:15p			
12:30p			
12:45p			
1:00p	Peters, Anthony		
1:15p	Peters, Monica C		
1:30p	Peters, Zach		
1:45p			
2:00p	Bordon, John		
2:15p	Gooding, Charles		
2:30p	Simpson, Tanus J		
2:45p	Clinger, Wallace		
3:00p	Jasper, Stephanie L		
3:15p	Jacks, Theodore		
3:30p			
3:45p			
4:00p	Karvel, Jessica C		
4:15p	Doogan, James		
4:30p	Zimmerman, Anthony		
4:45p	Palmdale, Timothy		

Printed 7/14/2008 1:16 pm

(Note that on these two examples, lunch has been slotted from 11:00–1:00. This may be to allow time for other office activities or physician scheduling needs.) The difference between the Grid View and the List View is that the Grid View shows the columns and time slots. The List View displays only a list of patients with their appointment times.

Tip: When moving between the Appointment window and MediSoft window, minimize the Appointment window. Doing so makes it easier to see the information you are trying to view.

The Patient Recall List

Many patients need follow-up appointments in a week, month, or year. MediSoft allows the user to create and edit a **patient recall list**. In the MediSoft window (*not* the appointment book window), pull down the Lists menu and select Patient Recall. The following window will appear:

To add a patient to the recall list, click the New button. The following dialog box will be displayed:

Fill in the information by making choices from the drop-down lists. After you select the chart number, MediSoft fills in the patient's name and phone numbers. You need to choose the procedure and type the message. (You can search by Procedure Code by using the up/down arrow or typing the procedure name.) Make sure you select the "Call" recall status at the bottom of the window.

Click on the Save button. Next click on Lists, go to Patient Recall and ensure that what you entered appears on the recall list.

Summary

- Launch the program by double-clicking on the MediSoft icon on the desktop. MediSoft's window resembles any other window, containing a title bar, menu bar, toolbar, and so on.
- Office Hours, which is a separate application program, can be launched by double-clicking on the icon on the desktop or from within MediSoft. It is MediSoft's appointment scheduler program.
- MediSoft uses two dates: the Windows system date and the MediSoft date.
- Appointments are made by choosing a provider, double-clicking the time of the appointment, and entering some information. (Information you have already entered in another part of the program can be linked easily without having to retype the data.)

- Breaks can be entered by clicking on the Break icon and filling in the relevant information.
- Repeat appointments are easily made using Search and Search Again.
- All appointments, breaks, and so on are color coded on the calendar.
- MediSoft allows the user to create a patient recall list with the dates and reasons for recall.

Review Exercises

Hands-on Exercises

1. Enter a coffee break every day at 10:00 AM for 15 minutes. Print the appointment list for today and tomorrow.
2. Enter an appointment for Dwight Again for one week from October 11, 2008 (on October 18, 2008). Print the appointment list for the week of October 12–October 18, 2008.
3. Choose a different provider from the provider list, and make three monthly appointments (starting with today's date) for Andrew Austin. Print the appointment lists for today, one month from today, and two months from today.
4. Change the MediSoft date to October 14, 2008. Make an appointment for 9:00 AM that day for Jay Brimley.

Change the date back to today's date. Make an appointment for Jane Doe for 8:45 AM. Print the appointment schedule for October 14, 2008, and for today.

Fill-in Questions

1. In MediSoft, _____ keys work as global commands, that is, they work from any part of the program.
2. The _____ menu contains options that allow the user to manage finances, insurance claims, and appointments, and to enter patient, diagnosis, procedure, and case information.

CHAPTER FIVE

ENTERING PATIENT AND CASE INFORMATION—A HANDS-ON APPROACH

■✗ Chapter Outline

- Patients and Cases
  - Entering and Editing Patient and Case Information
    - Jenna Green: Adding a New Patient with Medicare
    - Kathy Patel: Entering a New Uninsured Patient
    - Tonya Brown: Entering a Patient with Private Insurance
    - Jenna Green: Entering Case Information for a Patient with Medicare
    - Jenna Green: Editing Patient Information
    - Jenna Green: Adding a New Case for an Established Patient
    - Kathy Patel: Adding a Case for an Uninsured Patient
- Reports
  - Printing Patient Information
  - Printing Case Information
- A Note on Backing Up and Restoring Data
- Summary
- Review Questions
- Review Exercises

■✗ Learning Objectives

Upon completion of this chapter, the student will be able to:

- Understand what a case is.
- Enter, edit, and save patient files with several types of insurance.
- Enter, edit, and save cases for patients.
- Print reports on patient information (patient encounter forms and patient lists).
- Print case information.
- Back up data on a CD or flash drive and restore it on another computer.

▪️✖️ Key Terms

Assigned Provider	Custom Report	Primary Insurance
Back Up	Condition	Restore
Case Number	Insurance Carrier	Secondary Insurance
Chart Number	Patient List	Visit

Patients and Cases

Entering and Editing Patient and Case Information

When a new patient comes in for a scheduled appointment, the patient fills out forms with personal, health, insurance, and other information. The doctor enters diagnoses and procedures on the encounter form. All this information could be kept on paper. However, entering it into a computerized relational database such as MediSoft means that the information will be kept in an organized, easy-to-access fashion. Information is entered using on-screen forms; as you save it, it becomes part of a table in a relational database. If you edit and save a record on one form, that information is updated in other tables in which it appears. Entering information only once saves time and effort and guarantees the data is the same everywhere it appears.

We will start by entering patient and case information. MediSoft is an accounting program, and although we are starting with patients and cases, some of the information we enter has a bearing on what we do later, for example, entering transactions and handling claims. An insurance carrier is the company that insures a patient. The type of insurance a patient has—Medicare, private, managed care, or none—will affect other functions in the program. The first patient we will enter is Jenna Green; she is older than sixty-five and, therefore, has Medicare. The second patient we will enter is Kathy Patel, who just graduated from college; she is no longer under her parents' insurance policy and has only a part-time job. She cannot afford private insurance, so she has none. The last patient is Tonya Brown, whose medical insurance is one of her benefits as a full-time teacher. She has Aetna US Health Care for **primary insurance** and Blue Cross/Blue Shield as **secondary insurance**. Both are Preferred Provider Organizations (PPOs), which is a type of managed care. In the exercises that follow this chapter, you will enter a record for yourself. You have managed care, but the type you have is an HMO (Health Maintenance Organization).

JENNA GREEN: ADDING A NEW PATIENT WITH MEDICARE To enter Jenna Green, launch MediSoft, double-click the Patient Lists icon or select Patients/Guarantors and Cases from the Lists menu.

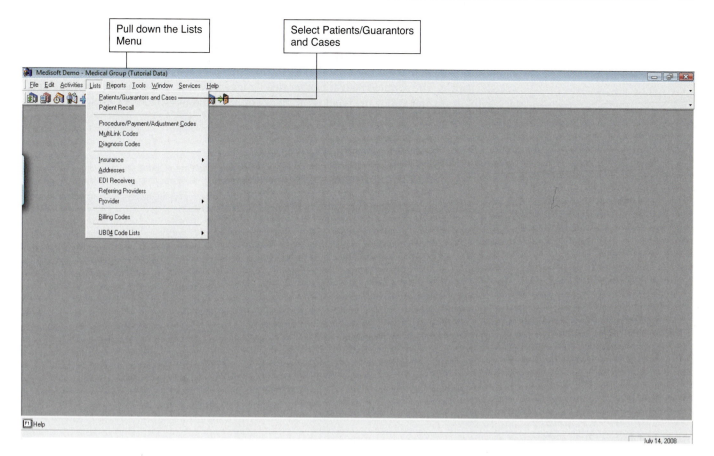

Make sure you are using the tutorial data. The following screen should appear:

The left pane contains a list of patients and information, including chart number, name, address, phone numbers, Social Security number, indication if signature is on file, patient type, gender, date of birth, provider, payment information, and employment data. However, to see all of this information, the user must scroll to the right. The right pane contains a list of cases for the selected patient. The selected patient is indicated by an arrowhead. **Case numbers** are assigned by MediSoft. At the top of the window are two circular buttons—one for Cases and one for Patients. Make sure Patient is selected.

Notice that this list is sorted by **chart number**. The chart number consists of the first three letters of the patient's last name, the first two letters of the first name, and three additional digits. You can indicate which field you want to search on, although the chart number is the default. To search for a patient, enter the first three letters of the patient's last name in the Search Box and press Enter. Patients with chart numbers matching your search term will be displayed.

At the bottom of the window are a series of command buttons.

Edit Patient allows you to see and change information in an existing patient's chart. New Patient and Delete Patient allow you to add a new patient and delete a patient, respectively. If the Case option button is chosen, these command buttons are modified to apply to cases instead of patients.

Prior to entering information on a patient, note that in MediSoft version 14, the user can set the program to hyphenate social security numbers by clicking file, program options, data entry, and clicking on auto format social security numbers.

- When you tab from the second address line, MediSoft brings you to the ZIP code. Fill in the ZIP. If MediSoft is familiar with that ZIP (if it appears previously), MediSoft will fill in the city and state for you. Otherwise you have to fill in this information yourself. Phone numbers can be entered without parentheses and hyphens; MediSoft automatically inserts them.

- Type all dates using eight digits (e.g., January 1, 2008 = 01012008).

    In MediSoft version 14, the user can enter additional information, including emergency contacts, cell phone and fax numbers, and e-mail address.

- After completing the form, click the Save button in the upper-right corner or press `F3` . MediSoft enters a chart number for you. MediSoft also checks for duplicate Social Security numbers.

    One other thing to keep in mind, as you enter information into the two tabbed areas (Patient Information tab and Other Information tab), you can either click on save once you have entered information in each tabbed area or you can wait until all of the information in both areas has been entered and then select save. Some individuals prefer to select save each time a tabbed area is completed to ensure that information is not accidently deleted or lost.

    Complete the following:

- Click on the New Patient option button or press F8. The following dialog box appears:

- Add the following data (maximize the window if you haven't already done so):
  - Tab over the chart number to the Last Name field.
  - With the insertion point in the Last Name field, type *Green*.
  - Tab to the First Name field and type *Jenna*.
  - Add the rest of the information (omitting chart number): Street Address—6060 Amsterdam Avenue, New York, NY, 10025, USA; Home Phone—2128646710 (no hyphens); Birth Date—11/20/1935 (eight-digit format); Sex—Female; Social Security Number—111223334 (no hyphens).

Look at the Patient List. Jenna Green is correctly placed in chart number order. (You will have to scroll to the left to see her name). You could click on the Other Information tab and add her provider, but there are other places to add the provider. We will add it when we add her new case information.

KATHY PATEL: ENTERING A NEW UNINSURED PATIENT Kathy Patel had been using her college's health services and her parents' insurance until graduation. Because her job is defined as part time, she has no health insurance. She calls the medical group practice to tell them she would like to become their patient but does not make an appointment at this time. They send her the forms she needs to fill out. She returns the completed paperwork, and a medical office worker enters the information into MediSoft's patient table in the practice's database.

To enter Kathy Patel as a patient, do the following:

- Pull down the Lists menu and select Patients/Cases and Guarantors. Press `F8` or the New Patient option button.
- Fill in the following information:

- Notice that when you enter the ZIP and press the Tab or Enter key, MediSoft fills in the city and state.

- Press the Save button or press `F3`.
- Press Enter. You will see Kathy Patel's name in the Patient List.
- Open her record and you will see the chart number MediSoft assigned.

Other Information Tab

```
Patient / Guarantor: Patel, Kathy                          [-] [□] [x]

Name, Address | Other Information |

Chart Number: PATKA000                                          [ Save ]

                                   Inactive [ ]                 [ Cancel ]

                                                                [ Help ]
  Last Name: [Patel]
 First Name: [Kathy]
Middle Name: [                        ]
     Street: [785 West End Avenue     ]                    [ Copy Address... ]
            [                          ]
       City: [New York      ]  State: [NY]                 [ Appointments ]
   Zip Code: [10025   ]  Country: [USA      ]
     E-Mail: [                         ]
       Home: [(212)234-5678]  Work: [(602)453-9988]
       Cell: [             ]  Fax:  [             ]
      Other: [             ]

 Birth Date: [6/12/1976  ▼]     Sex: [Female   ▼]
Birth Weight: [0          ]   Units: [         ▼]
Social Security: [        ]  Entity Type: [Person ▼]
```

- Now click on the Other Information tab and enter the information below. Make sure you enter *C* for cash. Each patient must have an assigned provider chosen from the drop-down list on the Other Information tab. Choose J.D. Mallard, MD, (JM) as the assigned provider. The Signature on File check box indicates whether or not the patient's signature is on file; check it so the patient does not have to sign each insurance form. All insurance companies that the provider represents require this box to be checked.

- Click the Save button or press [F3] .

TONYA BROWN: ENTERING A PATIENT WITH PRIVATE INSURANCE Tonya Brown is a full-time teacher at a public school with a strong faculty union. One of the negotiated benefits is medical coverage. She had a choice of plans and chose Aetna because all the health-care providers she visited were in the Aetna network of providers, as was the better hospital in her neighborhood. As a secondary insurer, she selected Blue Cross/Blue Shield.

Enter Tonya in the patient table by doing the following:

- Choose Patients/Guarantors and Cases.

- Click the New Patient option button at the bottom of the screen or press [F8] and fill in the

  following information. When you click on Save or press [F3] , MediSoft will assign a chart number (BROTO000), and take you back to the patient list.

- With Tonya Brown highlighted, click the Edit Patient option button.
- Click the Other Information tab and fill in the following:

- Click the Save button or press F3.

JENNA GREEN: ENTERING CASE INFORMATION FOR A PATIENT WITH MEDICARE Jenna called to make an appointment. Her reason for seeing the health-care provider is called a case. There can be more than one visit associated with one case. As long as the underlying **condition** remains the same, many visits constitute one case. And of course, there can be many different cases associated with one patient.

To add a new case for Jenna, do the following:

- Click on Jenna's record in the Patient List.
- Make sure the Case option button is chosen. Jenna's record will no longer be highlighted, but there will be an arrowhead next to it.
- Click the New Case option button at the bottom of the screen or press F8.

You will see the following tabbed dialog box with the Personal tab chosen and the name and guarantor filled in.

- Fill in the rest of the information.

- Click on Save or press F3; you will be told that there is no **assigned provider**. Click OK.
- Click on the Account tab.

Click on Account tab

- Click the down arrow in the Assigned Provider drop-down list box and select Melvin Morris.
- Click the down arrow in the Case Billing Code drop-down list box and choose *M* for Medicare.

- Click on the Save button or press F3.

NOTE: AS YOU GO THROUGH AND COMPLETE EACH OF THE TABBED DIALOG BOXES, YOU CAN EITHER CLICK THE SAVE BUTTON EACH TIME A TABBED AREA IS FILLED IN OR WAIT UNTIL ALL OF YOUR INFORMATION IS ENTERED. SOME RECOMMEND THAT YOU SAVE AS YOU GO SINCE THIS WILL ENSURE NO INFORMATION IS ACCIDENTLY DELETED. IF IN SAVING YOU ARE BROUGHT BACK TO THE LIST OF PATIENTS/CASES AND GUARANTORS, CLICK ON THE PATIENT YOU ARE ENTERING AND CLICK THE EDIT PATIENT COMMAND BUTTON. IF YOU ARE ENTERING A CASE, CLICK ON THE PATIENT, CLICK ON THE CASE OPTION BUTTON, AND CLICK ON THE EDIT CASE COMMAND BUTTON.

- Click on the Policy 1 tab and select Medicare from the Insurance 1 drop-down list. In the Policy Holder 1 tab, select the patient's name from the drop-down list. To save your information, again press F3 or click the Save button on the right side of your screen.

● Click on the Condition tab. The following dialog box appears:

● Fill in the information by typing in the date and making choices from drop-down lists for the other fields. Do not fill in anything in fields that are blank.

- Click the Save button or press F3.
- Click on the Diagnosis tab and fill in the diagnosis by clicking on the down arrow in the Principal Diagnosis drop-down list. You will have to either scroll through the choices until you see *Fracture, Finger* or click on the magnifying glass to open the search window. Click on Fracture, Finger. MediSoft fills in the code.
- Under Allergies and Notes, type *Allergic to aspirin.*
- Click the save button or press F3.

JENNA GREEN: EDITING PATIENT INFORMATION Once a patient is entered in the system, it is possible to change patient information. If Jenna calls to say she has moved to a new address, do the following:

- Pull down the Lists menu.
- Choose Patients/Guarantors and Cases.
- In the dialog box that opens, choose the Patient option button.

- Click on Jenna's record.

- Click on the Edit Patient option button at the bottom of the screen.

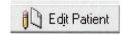

- Enter the new address: 123 Broadway.

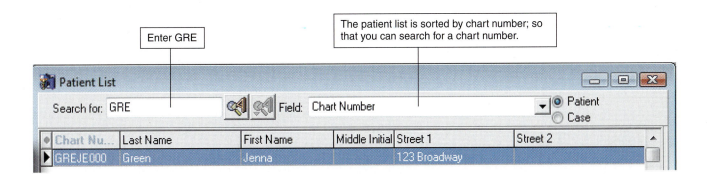

- Click the Save button or press F3.

Jenna has one follow-up appointment for her broken finger (two appointments for one case).

JENNA GREEN: ADDING A NEW CASE FOR AN ESTABLISHED PATIENT Several weeks later Jenna woke up with a sore throat and called the health-care provider to make an appointment. Pull down the Patient List, and make sure it is sorted by chart number. It is easy to find a patient by typing in the first three letters of the patient's last name. Enter *GRE* as a search term.

Once you have found the patient, do the following:

- Choose the Case option button. You could click on New Case; however, if you did that, you would have to reenter much of the same information that was already input for an earlier case on Jenna Green.

- Click on the Copy Case option button at the bottom of the screen. This will duplicate the information from Jenna Green's previous case.

Click copy case

- Now all you need to do is to change only the information that will be different for the new case you are creating.

The following dialog box will appear:

Do the following:

● Change the description to *sore throat*.

The case number will be assigned by MediSoft once the information is saved. All other information on this screen remains the same.

● Click the Save button or press F3.
● Click on the Diagnosis tab. The following screen appears:

● Click the down arrow in the Principal Diagnosis drop-down list and select *strep throat*.
● Click the Save button or press F3.
● Click the Condition tab.

- Type in the date 08042008 and choose *Illness* from the drop-down Illness Indicator list. Enter the first consultation date as 08042008. Enter dates unable to work from 8/4/2008 to 8/5/2008.

- Click the Save button or press F3.

Look at the Patient List by selecting the patient option button. Click on Jenna Green. You will see two cases associated with Jenna Green's name.

KATHY PATEL: ADDING A CASE FOR AN UNINSURED PATIENT Kathy Patel was jogging when she tripped and sprained her ankle. She called the practice to make an appointment. She had already filled out the patient information form and that data was entered. To add the case information, do the following:

- If not already open, launch MediSoft.
- Pull down the Lists menu and choose Patients/Cases and Guarantors.
- Select Kathy's record.
- Click on the Case option button.

- Click on the New Case option button [New Case] and fill in the following information on the personal page of the dialog box:

Case: PATKA000 Patel, Kathy [Sprained Ankle]

Condition | Miscellaneous | Medicaid and Tricare | Comment | EDI
Personal | Account | Diagnosis | Policy 1 | Policy 2 | Policy 3

Save
Cancel
Help

Case Number: 0

Description: Sprained Ankle   ☑ Cash Case
Global Coverage Until: ☑ Print Patient Statement
Guarantor: PATKA000   Patel, Kathy
Marital Status: Single   Student Status: Non-student

Eligibility...

Employment
Employer: BEA00   BeanSprout Express
Status: Part time
Retirement Date: Work Phone: (602)453-9988
Location: Extension:

Patient Information
Name: Patel, Kathy   Home Phone: (212)234-5678
Address: 785 West End Avenue   Work Phone: (602)453-9988
New York, NY   Cell Phone:
10025   Date of Birth: 6/12/1976

Case

- Click the Save button or press F3.

● Click on the Account tab and make sure the following information is entered:

- Click on the Diagnosis tab.
- Click the down arrow in the Principal Diagnosis drop-down list and select *sprained ankle.*
- Click the Save button or press F3.

- Click on the Condition tab and fill in the following information:

- Click the Save button or press F3.
- If an error message appears that says a provider has not been selected, select J.D. Mallard, MD, (JM) and press the Save button.

  Because she has no insurance, there is no other information to input.

Reports

Printing Patient Information

In MediSoft version 14, most printing is done from the Reports menu. To print a list of patients, do the following:

- Pull down the Reports menu and select **Custom Report** list.

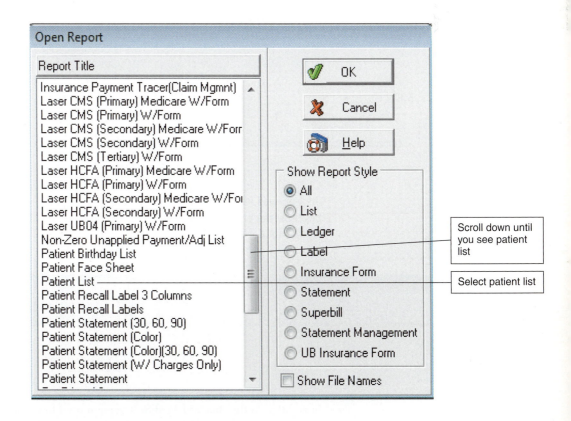

The following list will be displayed:

- Scroll down until you see Patient List and select it.
- Click OK.
- In the Print Report Where? dialog box, make sure Preview the Report on the Screen is selected and click Start.

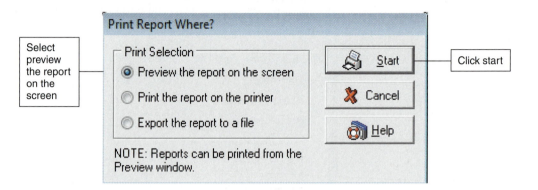

The next screen asks for the Range of Chart Numbers you want to print.

- Leave the range blank to print all records.

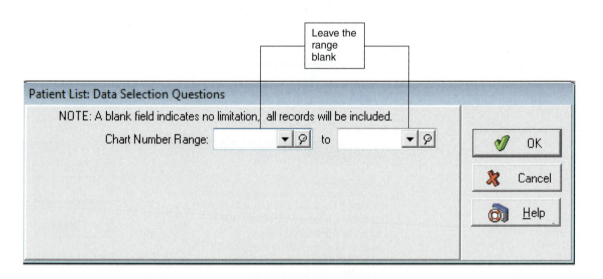

- Click OK. The first page you will see will be a cover sheet. Starting on the second page is the **Patient List**. To see the list of patients, press the arrow key at the top to go to the second page. Do not print it at this time. Print it only after completing all the Hands-on Exercises at the end of this chapter.

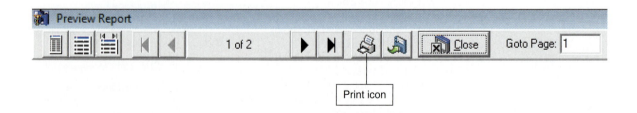

In addition to the standard MediSoft version used to teach MediSoft in training settings, there is a MediSoft Advanced version that provides additional functions. For instance, in MediSoft Advanced (version 14), you can print from almost any window.

Printing Case Information

The steps to print case information are very similar to the steps for printing patient information.

- Pull down the Reports menu and select Custom Report.
- Select Patient Face Sheet.
- Click OK.
- Select Preview the Report on the Screen.
- In the Data Range dialog box, using the drop-down list, enter the chart number for Jenna Green in both boxes. Click OK. To view Jenna's report, be sure and go to the second page of the report.
- Print the report only after completing the Hands-On Exercises.

A Note on Backing Up and Restoring Data

Unless you are using MediSoft Network Professional with a backup program, you may need to carry your MediSoft database from one computer to another. You can do this by **backing up** your files on a CD or flash drive and **restoring** them on another computer. You can back up your data by pulling down the File menu and selecting Backup Data.

A Backup Warning dialog box appears. Click OK.

In the Backup window, change the destination file path to reflect your drive. For example: Enter E:\.

Make sure you have a disk in the indicated drive before clicking Start Backup. Click Restore. Click Start. The following message will then appear: Backup file already exists. Do you want to replace it? Click Yes. A new message saying that the backup is complete will appear. Click OK. When MediSoft has finished backing up your data, the following window is displayed:

Click OK.

To view your existing backup files, go to File, View Backup Disks. The following window is displayed:

View Backup

Source Path:

E:\   Find

Existing Backup Files

mw7-15-2008.mbk

Password:

Original Data Path:

C:\MediData\Tutor\   View Backup

Backup Progress

0%   Close

File Progress

0%   Help

To access the data on the disk, for example, to work on it on another computer, you cannot simply open My Computer and click on the drive where the data is stored. It will not open the backup file. Instead, pull down the File menu and select Restore Data. Make sure you have your backup CD or flash drive inserted.

Medisoft Demo - Medical Group (Tutorial Data)

File Edit Activities Lists Reports Tools Windo

Open Practice...

New Practice...

Backup Data...

View Backup Disks...

Restore Data...

Backup Root Data...

Restore Root Data...

Set Program Date

Practice Information...

Program Options...

Security Setup...

Login/Password Management...

File Maintenance...

Exit   Alt+F4

The following warning will appear:

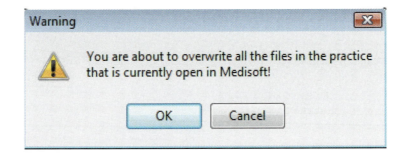

If you click OK, the following dialog box is displayed:

Once having made sure that the correct destination for the source disk is indicated, click the Start Restore button. When prompted that MediSoft is about to restore the file, click OK.

When the restore is finished, the following message is displayed on the screen:

Remember to always back up your data in case of accidental power loss, computer crash, etc.

Summary

- Profiles for patients with different types of insurance can be entered, edited, and saved on a patient form. As the records are saved, they become part of a patient list.
- A case is the condition for which a patient seeks treatment from a health-care provider. There can be several cases associated with one patient and several visits associated with one case.
- Case information, including condition, diagnoses, and insurance carriers, is entered in a multipage (tabbed) dialog box. As soon as it is saved, it becomes part of a case record for a patient.
- If you are using the standard MediSoft version, almost all printing is done from the Reports menu. There are many custom reports. You choose a report and fill in the range. To print all patients, leave the range blank. To print one patient, fill in that patient's chart number in both the "To" and "From" boxes. When using the MediSoft Advanced version, printing can be performed from almost any window.
- Data can be copied onto a CD or flash drive and restored on another computer.

Review Questions

1. MediSoft creates chart numbers using the first three letters of the patient's last name followed by the first two letters of the patient's first name, followed by three digits (000 if the patient is the only one with that name). What chart numbers would MediSoft create for the following patients?

   Loretta Washington _____

   Jennifer Ramirez _____

   David Cohen _____

   Edith Shah _____

   Debby Chin_____

2. Define the following terms.

   Case _____

   Carrier _____

   Medicare _____

   Guarantor _____

Review Exercises

Be sure to save each page of a tabbed dialog box by pressing 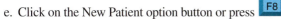 F3 or clicking on the save command button immediately after you fill in the information. You will be brought back to the list of patients/cases and guarantors. Click on the patient you are entering and click edit patient. If you are entering a case, click on the patient, click on the case option button, and click on edit case.

1. Enter a new patient with your own first and last names by doing the following:
   a. Launch MediSoft by double-clicking on its icon.
   b. Pull down the Lists menu.
   c. Select Patients/Guarantors and Cases.
   d. Make sure the Patient option button is selected.
   e. Click on the New Patient option button or press F8 .
   f. In the dialog box that opens, fill in your own information: your last and first names, address, date of birth, and so on.
   g. Click on the Other Information tab. Enter JM as your provider.
   h. Save the record. Look at the Patient List. Your name should be correctly placed in chart number order.

2. Add a case for yourself; you belong to a CIGNA HMO. Do the following:
   a. Pull down the Lists menu and select Patients/ Guarantors and Cases.
   b. Select yourself as the patient by clicking on your record.
   c. Click on the Case option button. Notice that your record is no longer selected, but there is a pointer next to it.
   d. Click on the New Case option button or press F8 . Note that MediSoft enters a case number.

   Of course your chart number will be made up of the letters of your last and first names.

e. Make sure you click on the Policy 1 tab and fill in the following. Your insurance is CIGNA.

f. Click on the Accounts tab. Make sure the Billing Code is *H* for HMO.

g. Click on the Diagnosis tab.

h. Click on the down arrow in the Principal Diagnosis drop-down list. Scroll down until you see *influenza*. Click on it.

i. Click on the Condition tab.

j. Fill in the Illness/Injury/LMP Date and First Consultation Date as today's date.

k. Click on the down arrow in the Illness Indicator drop-down list and select *illness.*

l. Click on the down arrow in the Death/Status drop-down list and select *Normal.*

m. In the Unable to Work field, fill in today's date in the from date and tomorrow's date as the to date.

n. After all of the information has been added for the case, click Save to save your entries. Look at the Patient List. Your name has a case associated with it.

3. Enter a new case for Tonya Brown.

a. Her personal information in the case dialog box is as follows:
   - The guarantor and case number are filled in by MediSoft. You may have to fill in employer and employment information.
   - Description: Bronchitis

- Marital Status: Single
- Student Status: Nonstudent

b. On the Account page, fill in her case billing code as *H* for HMO patient. Scroll down and enter treatment authorized through 9/1/2008.

c. On the diagnosis page, select *bronchitis* as the principal diagnosis.

d. On the condition page, fill in 8/15/2008, as the illness date, the illness indicator as *illness,* and the first consultation date as 8/18/2008. Tonya will be unable to work from 8/15/2008 to 8/19/2008.

e. On the Policy 1 page, choose Aetna from the Insurance 1 drop-down list and 9/1/2008, as the start date of the policy.

f. On the Policy 2 page, choose Blue Cross/Blue Shield 231 as the secondary insurer. Enter the policy number, group number, and policy date information below.

Be sure again, after you have entered all of the data for the case, that you click on Save to save your information.

4. Print the Patient List and the Patient Face Sheets for yourself, Jenna Green, Kathy Patel, and Tonya Brown.

See pages 61–62 for printing instructions. Remember, when you print the patient face sheets, each patient has to be printed as a separate report. Enter the chart number of the patient you want to print in the "From" and "To" drop-down lists.

Patient List

Happy Valley Medical Clinic
Patient List
7/15/2008

Chart	Name	CityLine	Phone
AGADW000	Dwight Again	Phoenix, AZ 85021	434-5777
AUSAN000	Andrew Austin	Tempe, AZ 85123	767-2222
BORJO000	John Bordon	Scottsdale, AZ 85777	(434)777-1234
BRIEL000	Elmo Brimley	Glendale, AZ 85382	(222)342-3444
BRIJA000	Jay Brimley	Glendale, AZ 85382	(222)342-3444
BRISU000	Susan Brimley	Glendale, AZ 85382	(222)342-3444
BROTO000	Tonya Brown	New York, NY 10025	(212)968-5874
CATSA000	Sammy Catera	Gilbert, 85001	227-7722
CLIWA000	Wallace Clinger	Washington, DC 11111	(254)222-9111
DOEJA000	Jane S. Doe	Mesa, AZ 85213	(480)999-9999
DOEJO000	John Doe	Mesa, AZ 85213	(480)999-9999
DOOJA000	James Doogan		
GOOCH000	Charles Gooding		
GREJE000	Jenna Green	New York, NY 10025	(212)864-6710
HARTO000	Tonya Hartman	Portland, OR 97532	847-6199
JACTH000	Theodore Jacks	Gilbert, AZ 85297	

Patient Face Sheet Jenna Green

Happy Valley Medical Clinic
Patient Face Sheet
7/15/2008

Patient Chart #: GREJE000   D.O.B: 11/20/1935   Age: 72
Patient Name: Jenna Green   Sex: Female
Street 1: 123 Broadway   SSN: 111-22-3334
Street 2:   Mar Status: Divorced
City: New York, NY 10025   S.O.F:
Phone: (212)864-6710   Assigned Provider:

Employer Name: Micro Mania Inc.
Street 1: 57 N. 103rd St.
City: Phoenix, AZ 85213
Phone: (602)746-2134

Case Information

Case Desc: Sore Throat   Diagnosis 1: 034.0
Last Visit: Diagnosis 2:
Referral: Diagnosis 3:
Guarantor Name: Jenna Green   Diagnosis 4:
Street 1: 123 Broadway

Kathy Patel's Patient Face Sheet

Happy Valley Medical Clinic
Patient Face Sheet
7/15/2008

Patient Chart #: PATKA000
Patient Name: Kathy Patel
Street 1: 785 West End Avenue
Street 2:
City: New York, NY 10025
Phone: (212)234-5678

D.O.B: 06/12/1976   Age: 32
Sex: Female
SSN:
Mar Status: Single
S.O.F: 7/14/2008
Assigned Provider: J.D. Mallard

Employer Name: Bean Sprout Express
Street 1: Old Town Mall
City: Scottsdale, AZ 85216
Phone: (602)453-9988

Case Information

Case Desc: Sprained Ankle
Last Visit:
Referral:
Guarantor Name: Kathy Patel
Street 1: 785 West End Avenue

Diagnosis 1: 845.00
Diagnosis 2:
Diagnosis 3:
Diagnosis 4:

Tonya Brown's Patient Face Sheet

Happy Valley Medical Clinic
Patient Face Sheet
8/11/2008

Patient Chart #: BROTO000
Patient Name: Tonya Brown
Street 1: 229 West 109th Street
Street 2:
City: New York, NY 10025
Phone: (212)968-5874

D.O.B: 06/14/1960   Age: 48
Sex: Female
SSN: 444-55-6677
Mar Status: Single
S.O.F: 7/14/2008
Assigned Provider: Melvin Morris

Employer Name: Tempe Elem. School Dist. 4
Street 1:
City: Tempe, AZ
Phone:

Case Information

Case Desc: Bronchitis
Last Visit:
Referral:
Guarantor Name: Tonya Brown
Street 1: 229 West 109th Street

Diagnosis 1: 490.0
Diagnosis 2:
Diagnosis 3:
Diagnosis 4:

Your Patient Face Sheet

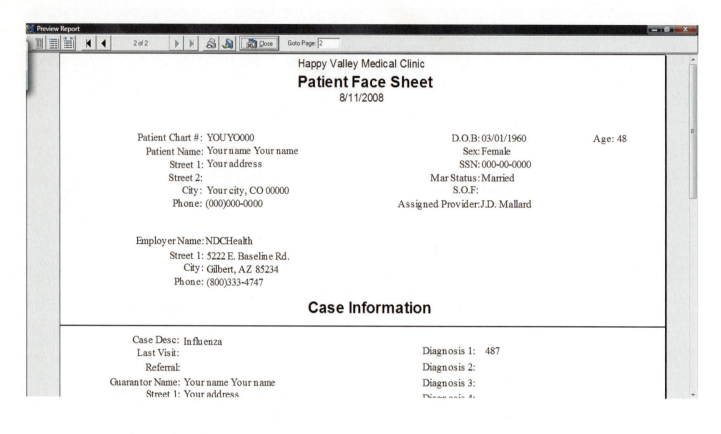

CHAPTER SIX

AN INTRODUCTION TO TRANSACTION ENTRY AND CLAIM MANAGEMENT

Chapter Outline

- Transaction Entry
  - Entering Transactions: Charges
  - Entering Transactions: Payments and Adjustments
- Claim Management
  - Printing a Primary Claim Summary
- Entering Deposits
- Quick Ledger and Quick Balance
- Summary
- Review Exercises

Learning Objectives

Upon completion of this chapter, the student will:

- Be able to define *transaction*.
- Understand transaction entry.
- Be able to enter, edit, and apply payments and charges and save this information.
- Understand claim management.
- Know how to create and print claims.
- Check the status of claims.
- Understand how to apply payments to charges.
- Be able to print a Deposit List report.
- Know how to check on a patient's billing status using Quick Ledger and Quick Balance.

Key Terms

Adjustment

Allowed Amount

Batches

Case Number

Charge

Chart Number

Custom Report

Deposit List

Patient Face Sheet

Patient Statement

Payment

Primary Claim Summary

Procedure

Quick Balance

Quick Ledger

Walkout Receipt

Transaction Entry

Once a patient is established and has at least one case associated with her, transactions must be entered and claims sent to the insurance carrier (or bills to the patient).

A transaction can be a charge to the patient's account, a payment made by an insurance company or the patient, or an adjustment to the patient's account (adjustments are discussed in the next section).

Entering Transactions: Charges

In MediSoft version 14, to enter a transaction pull down the Activities menu and choose Enter Transactions or simply click the Activities icon. The following dialog box appears:

Scroll down so you can see the entire page. As you can see, there are two sections to this window. The top portion allows you to enter charges. The lower portion allows you to enter payments and adjustments.

To enter a new charge for Jenna Green, do the following:

- Pull down the Chart drop-down list and select Jenna Green's chart number.

- Pull down the Case Number drop-down list and select *Sore Throat* as the case. Your dialog box should appear similar to the following:

- Click New (you are entering a new transaction) then click on the first blank line under the word *Date.*
- Use the drop-down list to select the correct date.
- Click in the Procedure box. Use the drop-down list to select the correct CPT code.

> NOTE: EACH PROCEDURE HAS A CPT CODE. SOME CODES ALSO HAVE MODIFIERS MADE UP OF ONE OR TWO DIGITS. MODIFIERS ALLOW A MORE DETAILED DESCRIPTION OF THE PROCEDURE. NOTE THE MULTILINK COMMAND BUTTON. MULTILINK CODES ARE GROUPS OF CPT CODES THAT RELATE TO ONE ACTIVITY. THE MULTILINK LETS YOU USE ONE ACCESS CODE TO ENTER THE ENTIRE GROUP OF CODES AT ONCE IN **TRANSACTION ENTRY**. FOR EXAMPLE, IF YOU PERFORM PHYSICAL EXAMINATIONS AND HAVE THE SAME GROUP OF PROCEDURES AND CHARGES EACH TIME (SUCH AS A GENERAL HEALTH SCREEN, URINALYSIS, AND AN EKG), YOU CAN INCLUDE EACH OF THE PROCEDURES IN A SINGLE MULTILINK AND GIVE IT AN IDENTIFYING CODE NAME. USING MULTILINK CODES SAVES TIME.

- Click on the Amount box, and MediSoft will automatically fill in the price charged by the practice.
- Ensure that the Diag 1 box is filled in with the diagnosis.
- Ensure that the correct provider is selected in the Provider box.
- The amount allowed by the insurance company for the procedure is called the Allowed Amount. This information in the Allowed Amount tab will appear once the transaction has been entered and saved. Medicare, for example, allows $9.00 for a strep culture for which

the practice charges $15.00. The $6.00 is an adjustment to the patient's account. Once you return to the transaction entry screen, the allowed amount will appear.

Entering Transactions: Payments and Adjustments

It is important to document in the transaction record adjustments and payments. This is done in the Payment, Adjustment, and Comments area.

On Jenna Green's transactions, we must show that Medicare will pay $9.00 for the step culture and that an adjustment of $6.00 must be made to the account.

ENTERING THE PAYMENT To enter the payment amount to the allowed amount, follow these steps:

- Click on New in the Payments, Adjustments, and Comments section.
- Click on the Date, and enter the date of the patient's visit (8/4/2008).
- Indicate the Payment or Adjustment Code in the next box by finding the code and description in the drop-down list (MP—Medicare-Payment).
- Next select the group/individual who made the payment as indicated in the drop-down list (Medicare-Primary).
- Write in a description of the payment, such as Medicare Payment.
- Ensure the correct provider is listed correctly.
- Enter the payment ($9.00) in the Amount box.

- If a check number is applicable, note it.

		Date	Pay/Adj Code	Who Paid	Description	Provider	Amount	Check Number	Unapplied
		8/4/2008	MP	Medicare -Primary	Medicare Payment	MM	-9.00		$0.00
▶		8/4/2008	MED ADJ	Medicare -Primary	Medicare Writeoff	MM	-6.00		$0.00

Payments, Adjustments, And Comments:

🔲 Apply   🔲 New   🔲 Delete   🔲 Note

☑ Calculate Totals   🔲 Update All   🔲 Print Receipt   🔲 Print Claim   🔲 Close   🔲 Save Transactions

F1 Help   F2 MultiLink   F3 Save   F5 Note   F7 Ledger   Esc Cancel   F11 Quick Balance

- At the end of the first line, choose New.

ENTERING THE ADJUSTMENT

- Enter the same date (8/4/2008).
- In Payment/Adjustment Code box, select MED ADJ (Medicare write-off adjustment) from the drop-down list.
- The group/individual who paid (Medicare-Primary) should be indicated in the next field.
- The description of the adjustment, if any, would be entered next.
- Ensure the correct provider is listed.
- Enter the adjustment amount ($6.00) in the Amount box.
- If a check number is applicable, note it.

Once all of your information has been entered press the Apply button on the left hand side of the window. Don't press the Save Transactions button yet. Procedure charges and payments are linked through the apply payment to charges dialog box. A dialog box appears where you can enter the adjustment amount in the payment box. Once you have done so you can close the Apply Payment to Charges window.

Apply Adjustment to Charges

Adjustment
For: Green, Jenna

Unapplied
0.00

Date From	Document	Procedure	Charge	Balance	This Adjust.
8/4/2008	0808050000	87072	15.00	0.00	-6.00

There is 1 charge entry.   🔲 Close   🔲 Help

Note that on your transaction window that the $9.00 has not been applied. Click the Apply button and enter the amount of $9.00. Once you have entered the $9.00 in the payment box you can again close the Apply Payment to Charges window.

After all of your payment/adjustment information has been entered, click the Save Transactions button. In the section that shows the patients total charges and payments, the following should appear.

To create a new transaction for Jenna's fractured finger, click on the New button and fill in the relevant information.

You can print the claim by clicking on the Print Claim button. After filling in all transactions for Jenna, you can see each of them on the transaction screen by clicking on the drop-down list where Cases are indicated. You can also see them listed in a patient statement: Click Reports, Patient Statements, Start; fill in Green's chart number for the beginning and end of the range; and print.

Claim Management

You can see the billing status of your claims by printing a Primary Claim Summary. Click on the Reports menu and click Custom Report List. Select Primary Claim Summary. Click OK. Click Start. Fill in only the Claim Number Range (1–9) and click OK.

Primary Claim Summary: Data Selection Questions

NOTE: A blank field indicates no limitation, all records will be included.

Claim Primary Billing Date Range: [   ] to [   ]

Claim Number Range: [1   ] to [9   ]

Chart Number Range: [   ] to [   ]

✔ OK
✖ Cancel
Help

Preview Report — 2 of 2 — Close — Goto Page: 2

Happy Valley Medical Clinic
Primary Claim Summary
1/29/2009

Claim #	Batch #	Chart Number	Date Billed	Claim Status	Billed To	Claim Total
1	1	SIMTA000	12/03/2002	Sent	Aetna	396.00
2	2	AGADW000	11/21/2002	Done	Medicare	150.00
3	4	BRIJA000	03/25/2002	Sent	Cigna	95.00
4	5	BRISU000	12/05/2002	Done	Cigna	60.00
5	0	WAGJE000	06/01/2002	Sent	Blue Cross Blue Shield 231	105.00
6	0	YOUMI000		Ready to Send	U.S. Tricare	85.00
7	7	AGADW000	12/06/2002	Sent	Medicare	105.00
8	8	DOEJA000	12/06/2002	Done	Medicaid	160.00
9	9	JONSU000	04/04/2002	Done	FHP Health Plan	335.00

Be sure to save your work often.

Printing a Primary Claim Summary

You may now print a Primary Claim Summary for Jenna by doing the following:

- Pull down the Reports menu and choose Custom Report List.
- Select Primary Claim Summary.
- Click OK.

- Fill in GREJE000 in both the chart number range dialog boxes.

Primary Claim Summary: Data Selection Questions

NOTE: A blank field indicates no limitation, all records will be included.

Claim Primary Billing Date Range: [   ] ▼ to [   ] ▼

Claim Number Range: [   ] ▼ 𝒫 to [   ] ▼ 𝒫

Chart Number Range: [GREJE000] ▼ 𝒫 to [GREJE000] ▼ 𝒫

✓ OK

✗ Cancel

🛟 Help

- Click OK.
- You can see the status of the claim and print it. (Be sure to look on page 2 of the report to view the summary information).

Preview Report

2 of 2   ▶ ▶| Close   Goto Page: 2

Happy Valley Medical Clinic
Primary Claim Summary
8/6/2008

Claim #	Batch #	Chart Number	Date Billed	Claim Status	Billed To	Claim Total
10	0	GREJE000		Ready to Send	Medicare	30.00
11	0	GREJE000		Ready to Send	Medicare	15.00

On this list, both claims are ready to send.

To enter a new transaction for Tonya Brown, do the following:

- Click on the Transactions Entry icon or pull down the Activities menu and select Enter Transactions.
- Using the drop-down list, select the Chart number of the patient BROTO000.
- In the Charges Section, select New to enter the information for the new transaction. Fill in the procedure by clicking on the down-arrow in the Procedure drop-down list and selecting x-ray chest, 2 views. Once the procedure is filled in, MediSoft fills in the charge.

To indicate that a payment of $42.40 has been received from Aetna, you need to fill in the date of the payment (8/15/2008) and the code to indicate where the payment has originated (AP). Once the code has been selected, MediSoft will fill in Who Paid. If there is any description of the payment, it should be entered.

In this case, enter the word *Check* and the check number. Enter the amount paid and save your transaction.

- Click the Apply button and the following dialog box will appear:

Apply Payment to Charges							
Payment From: 1						Unapplied	-42.40
For: Brown, Tonya							
Date From	Document	Procedure	Charge	Balance	Payor Total	This Payment	Complete
8/15/2008	0808110000	71020	53.00	53.00	0.00	0.00	

☑ Automatically check the Complete column
There is 1 charge entry.

Close   Help

- In the Apply Payment to Charges box, fill in 42.40 as the payment.

Apply Payment to Charges							
Payment From: 1						Unapplied	0.00
For: Brown, Tonya							
Date From	Document	Procedure	Charge	Balance	Payor Total	This Payment	Complete
8/15/2008	0808110000	71020	53.00	10.60	-42.40	-42.40	✓

☑ Automatically check the Complete column
There is 1 charge entry.

Close   Help

- Click the Close button (at bottom of this box). You will notice in the upper right of the transaction window, where charges, adjustments, and other items are listed, that the Account Total is now zero.
- Once the payment has been entered, print the claim by clicking the Print Claim icon.

Note that Tonya's secondary insurance, BC/BS, will pay $8.48. Notice that after you choose BCBS Payment, when you tab to the next box, the default is set for Aetna. You must use the drop-down menu and choose BCBS 231. When you are done entering your applied amount, click on the Update All button to see all the changes. The account total will be $2.12, which is the patient's responsibility.

Save the transaction. The patient is billed for the remainder after the check and explanation of benefits (EOB) are received from BC/BS.

On your own, enter a transaction for yourself by pulling down the Activities menu and entering your own chart number.

- Fill in the required information as shown in the following figure.

Be sure to apply your payments and save your entry so you can see that the HMO (Cigna) paid the whole bill. Notice that the account total in the upper right corner is zero.

- Print the Patient Face Sheet. The Patient Face Sheet provides you detailed information on the patient and the case.

Preview Report

2 of 2   Close   Goto Page: 2

Happy Valley Medical Clinic
Patient Face Sheet
8/11/2008

Patient Chart #: YOUYO000	D.O.B: 03/01/1960 Age: 48
Patient Name: Your name Your name	Sex: Female
Street 1: Your address	SSN: 000-00-0000
Street 2:	Mar Status: Married
City: Your city, CO 00000	S.O.F:
Phone: (000)000-0000	Assigned Provider: J.D. Mallard

Employer Name: NDCHealth
Street 1: 5222 E. Baseline Rd.
City: Gilbert, AZ 85234
Phone: (800)333-4747

Case Information

Case Desc: Influenza	Diagnosis 1: 487
Last Visit: 8/11/2008	Diagnosis 2:
Referral:	Diagnosis 3:
Guarantor Name: Your name Your name	Diagnosis 4:
Street 1: Your address	
City: Your city, CO 00000	
Phone: (000)000-0000	
SSN: 000-00-0000	

Ins Co #: CIG00	Insured 1 Name: Your name Your name
Insurance 1: Cigna	Street 1: Your address
Street 1: 2525 Big Bucks Ln.	Street 2:
Street 2:	Phone: (000)000-0000
City: Mesa, AZ 85438	D.O.B.: 03/01/1960 Sex: Female
Phone: 234-5678	Policy Number: 232455
Ins-Start: 2/15/2008	Group Number: 54
End:	

Because Kathy Patel has no insurance, a claim does not have to be generated for her. She is handed a bill at the end of a visit, pays it, and is given a walkout receipt.

To see the status of all of your office's insurance claims, pull down the Activities menu and select Claim Management.

Medisoft Demo - Medical Group (Tutorial Data) - [Claim Management]

File   Edit   Activities   Lists   Reports   Tools   Window   Services   Help

Search: Sort By: List Only...   Change Status

Claim Number	Chart Number	Insurance Carrier 1	Status 1	Media 1	Batch Number 1	Primary Billing Date	EMC Receiver 1	Insurance Carrier 2	Status 2	Media 2	Batch Number 2	Secondary Billing Date	EMC Receiver 2	Insurance Carrier 3	Status
1	SIMTA000	AET00	Sent	Paper	1	12/3/2002					0				
2	AGADW000	MED01	Done	Paper	2	11/21/2002		AET00	Sent	Paper	3	12/4/2002			
3	BRIJA000	CIG00	Sent	Paper	4	3/25/2002		BLU01	Sent	Paper	4	3/25/2002	NAT00		
4	BRISU000	CIG00	Done	Paper	5	12/5/2002		BLU00	Sent	Paper	6	1/16/2002	NAT00		
5	WAGJE000	BLU00	Sent	EDI	0	6/1/2002	NAT00				0				
6	YOUMI000	US000	Ready to Send	Paper	0						0				
7	AGADW000	MED01	Sent	Paper	7	12/6/2002					0				
10	GREJE000	MED01	Ready to Send	Paper	0						0				
11	GREJE000	MED01	Ready to Send	Paper	0						0				
12	BROTO000	AET00	Ready to Send	Paper	0			BLU00	Ready to Send	Paper	0			NAT00	
13	AGADW000	MED01	Ready to Send	Paper	0			AET00	Ready to Send	Paper	0				
14	BORJO000	BLU01	Ready to Send	EDI	0		NAT00				0				
15	BRIJA000	CIG00	Ready to Send	Paper	0			BLU01	Ready to Send	EDI	0			NAT00	
16	DOOJA000	MED00	Ready to Send	Paper	0						0				
17	YOUYO000	CIG00	Ready to Send	Paper	0						0				

Edit   Create Claims   Print/Send   Reprint Claim   Claims Manager   Delete   Close

F1 Help   F9 Edit   Del Delete

The screen shows the status of every claim. The claims are organized in **batches** according to when they were created. The status of a claim includes the following:

- Whether it was submitted on paper or electronically
- Whether it is ready to send or has been sent to the primary insurer
- The response from the primary insurer
- Whether or not it is ready to send or has been sent to the secondary insurer

Each task has a date associated with it. You can view these items by using the scroll bar at the bottom of the screen.

We have been creating claims from the transaction entry window; however, you can create claims another way—by clicking on the Create Claims button at the bottom of the Deposits and Payments window. This window, though, is available only if you are using MediSoft Advanced version 14.

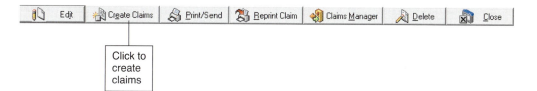

Click to create claims

Claims can also be printed, sent, reprinted, or deleted using these command buttons.

Entering Deposits

Payments must be deposited. As discussed earlier in this chapter, in MediSoft, payments can be applied when entering transactions. In MediSoft Advanced, deposits can be entered and a list of deposits can be creating by pulling down the Activities menu and selecting Enter Deposits and Payments. This action results in the appearance of the following dialog box:

Deposit List

Deposit Date: 9/8/2008 ☑ Show All Deposits ☐ Show Unapplied Only   Sort By: Date-Description   Detail...

Deposit Date	Description	Payor Name	Payor Type	Payment	Unapplied
6/13/2002	0206130000	Blue Cross Blue Shield 231	Insurance	84.00	0.00
8/22/2002	0208220000	Wagnew, Jeremy	Patient	22.00	0.00
12/3/2002	0212030000	Simpson, Tanus J	Patient	10.00	0.00
12/4/2002		Medicare	Insurance	119.00	0.00
12/5/2002		Zimmerman, Anthony	Patient	188.00	0.00
12/6/2002	0212060000	Doe, Jane S	Patient	10.00	0.00
12/11/2002		Medicaid	Insurance	56.00	0.00
12/27/2002		Simpson, Tanus J	Patient	25.00	25.00
4/4/2003		Aetna	Insurance	200.00	200.00
8/3/2003		Blue Cross Blue Shield 225	Insurance	55.00	55.00
9/29/2003		Cigna	Insurance	125.00	125.00
12/22/2003	0312220000	Medicaid	Insurance	EOB Only	0.00
12/22/2003	0312220000	Austin, Andrew	Patient	10.00	10.00
12/22/2003	0312220000	Cigna	Insurance	200.00	0.00
12/22/2003	0312220000	Austin, Andrew	Patient	10.00	0.00
12/22/2003	0312220000	Austin, Andrew	Patient	25.00	0.00

Edit   New   Apply   Print   Delete   Export   Close

BEWARE that it is critical to make sure you are working with the advanced version wherever this is noted in this textbook. If the advanced version is not used when indicated, you will not be able to perform the described tasks.

Quick Ledger and Quick Balance

Another function available in only MediSoft Advanced is a quick summary of a patient's procedures or billing and payment status. This can be done by pulling down the Activities menu and selecting Patient Ledger. Once the patient's chart number is selected from the drop-down list the following window will appear:

Print command button

It can be printed by clicking on the Print icon on the bottom of the screen.

If you simply want the patient's balance, pull down the Activities menu and select Quick Balance. Enter the chart number of the patient, and the following will appear:

This can be printed by clicking on the Print button.

Summary

- A transaction is a charge, payment, or adjustment to a patient account.
- A claim is a bill to an insurance carrier.
- Deposits are automatically entered on the deposit list when a payment is applied to a charge.
- The Quick Ledger shows you a summary of a patient's procedures and billing and payment status.
- The Quick Balance function shows a patient's balance.

Review Exercises

1. On your own, edit Dwight Again's transaction record to record an additional $24.65 payment from Medicare today. Print the deposit report; the last entry should be a check from Medicare for $24.65. Start by pulling down the Activities menu and selecting Enter Transactions. Pull up Dwight Again's chart and apply the payment in the Payments, Adjustments, and Comments area. Once the payment has been applied, save the transaction and close out of the transaction window. Go into Reports and print a patient statement on Dwight Again that shows the Medicare payment as seen in the following example:

Happy Valley Medical Clinic
5222 E. Baseline Rd.
Gilbert, AZ 85234
(800)333-4747

Statement Date	Page
1/29/2009	1

Dwight Again
1742 N. 83rd Ave.
Phoenix, AZ 85021

Chart Number
AGADW000

Date	Document	Description	Case Number	Amount
			Previous Balance:	0.00
Patient: Dwight Again		Chart #: AGADW000		
Case Description: Broken Hand		Date of Last Payment: 1/29/2009	Amount: -24.65	
9/3/2002	0209030000	X-Ray, Hand, Min 3 Views	2	45.00
9/3/2002	0209030000	Office Visit Est. Patient EEL	2	60.00
Patient: Dwight Again		Chart #: AGADW000		
Case Description: Back Pain		Date of Last Payment: 1/29/2009	Amount: -24.65	
11/21/2002	0211210000	Office Visit Est. Patient EEL	17	60.00
11/21/2002	0211210000	X-Ray, Spinal, Complete	17	80.00
11/21/2002	0211210000	Hot/Cold Pack Therapy	17	10.00
12/4/2002	0211210000	Medicare Payment	17	-48.00
12/4/2002	0211210000	Medicare Payment	17	-63.00
12/4/2002	0211210000	Medicare Payment	17	-8.00
12/4/2002	0211210000	Comment	17	0.00
3/9/2007	0703090000	Office Visit Est. Patient EEL	17	60.00
1/29/2009	0901290000	Medicare Payment	17	-24.65

Total Charges	Total Payments	Total Adjustments	Balance Due
$315.00	-$143.65	$0.00	171.35

CHAPTER SEVEN

ELECTRONIC MEDIA CLAIMS

Chapter Outline

- Submitting Electronic Media Claims
- Electronic Claim Management
- Electronic Transfer of Funds
- Reports Provided by Clearinghouses
- Summary
- Review Exercises

Learning Objectives

Upon completion of this chapter, the student will:

- Understand the process of submitting electronic claims.
- Know what information must be in place before an electronic claim is submitted.
- Understand the function of a clearinghouse.
- Appreciate the differences between paper claims and electronic claims.

Key Terms

Electronic Data Interchange (EDI)

Electronic Funds Transfer (EFT)

Electronic Remittance Advice (ERA)

National Provider Identifier (NPI)

NOTE: PLEASE NOTE THAT THIS CHAPTER IS FOR THE STUDENT'S INFORMATION ONLY. ALTHOUGH THE STUDENTS CAN RETRIEVE THE INFORMATION USING MEDISOFT, THESE TASKS CANNOT BE PERFORMED IN A CLASSROOM SETTING BECAUSE THE STUDENT DOES NOT HAVE ACCESS TO A CLEARINGHOUSE OR ANY INSURANCE COMPANY. THE ELECTRONIC CLAIM CAN BE SUBMITTED ONLY IN A REAL HEALTH-CARE OFFICE SETTING.

Submitting Electronic Media Claims

Claims can be submitted to insurance carriers either on paper or electronically as an electronic media claim (EMC). The way this is done varies regionally. Advantages to submitting claims electronically include elimination of paperwork, postage costs, carrier handling times (thereby improving cash flow by decreasing payment times from about twenty-six days to fourteen days). Errors are reduced also by eliminating manual keying and using system edits.

A health-care provider's office may choose to submit electronic claims directly to an insurer or through a clearinghouse (a business that collects claims from many offices and forwards them to the patient's insurance carriers).

Several tasks must be completed by the user before electronic claims can be submitted.

The information for patients, Electronic Data Interchange (EDI) receivers, insurance carriers, providers, and referring providers must be entered. To access the following lists, pull down the Lists menu and choose the appropriate option. Any of these lists can be edited or amended by the user.

MediSoft's tutorial includes a list of patients.

The tutorial database also has a table of EMC receivers set up.

A list of insurance carriers is included as well.

The tutorial database also contains a list of providers.

In addition, a referring provider list is included in the tutorial. The user can edit this list and add a new provider by clicking on the New button near the bottom of the window. Fill in the following information:

Click Save and Jane Smith's name will appear on the provider list.

code	last name	first name	middle initial	credentials	street 1	str
CAR00	Carlson	Carl			5226 E. Baseline Rd.	
PIE00	Pierce	Hawkeye		M.D.		
SMI00	Smith	Jane		MD	123 Broadway	
TRA00	Trapper	John		M.D.		

Electronic Claim Management

Although as a student you cannot create electronic claims, you can look at the claim management screen and see the various types of claim submissions. Pull down the Activities menu and select Claim Management.

Claim Number	Chart Number	Insurance Carrier 1	Status 1	Media 1	Batch Number 1	Primary Billing Date	EMC Receiver 1	Insurance Carrier 2	Status 2	Media 2	Ba
1	SIMTA000	AET00	Sent	Paper	1	12/3/2002					
2	AGADW000	MED01	Done	Paper	2	11/21/2002		AET00	Sent	Paper	
3	BRIJA000	CIG00	Sent	Paper	4	3/25/2002		BLU01	Sent	Paper	
4	BRISU000	CIG00	Done	Paper	5	12/5/2002		BLU00	Sent	Paper	
5	WAGJE000	BLU00	Sent	EDI	0	6/1/2002	NAT00				
6	YOUMI000	US000	Ready to Send	Paper	0						
7	AGADW000	MED01	Sent	Paper	7	12/6/2002					
10	GREJE000	MED01	Ready to Send	Paper	0						

To submit claims electronically, you and the insurance carrier need a modem.

Electronic Transfer of Funds

Electronic claims are usually paid by electronic funds transfer (EFT). The funds transfer can be accompanied by an electronic remittance advice (ERA), explaining the response to the claim. It is similar to the explanation of benefits (EOB) that accompanies the response to a paper claim but lists multiple patients for multiple doctors.

Electronic claims require the patient's first and last names, signature on file, the insured's policy and group numbers, dates and places of service, diagnoses, procedures, charges, and units of service. Provider information must include signature on file, full name, PIN, address, and phone number. The practice information must include the practice name.

As of May 28, 2008, the Medicare National Provider Identifier (NPI) is required for all HIPAA Standard Transactions. On all HIPAA electronic transactions and paper claims, the NPI must be used in the primary and secondary provider fields.

Reports Provided by Clearinghouses

When using MediSoft, transmitting insurance claims electronically can be done through the use of a clearinghouse such as RelayHealth Clearinghouse. A clearinghouse offers various reports that indicate if all the necessary information is included and accurate on the submitted claims. The following is an example of one type of report provided by the RelayHealth Clearinghouse:

```
                        TSH 277 CLAIM STATUS REJECT REPORT          PAGE:     1
     CPA425.02                                                       MM/DD/CCYY
                                                                     15:56:37

     CONTROL #:       112049999
     DATE/TIME:       03/02/05  15:56
     PROD/TEST:       P
     ORIGINATOR APPLICATION TRANS ID:        149999
     TRANSACTION SET CREATION DATE:          MM/DD/CCYY
     CLIENT ID/NAME:          009999 PHYSICAINS, INC
     SUBMITTER ID/NAME:       929999 PHYSICIANS INC
     ------------------------------------------------------------------------
     SUBSCR NAME:  PAUL JOHNSON
     PATIENT NAME: POLLY JOHNSON
     PAYER ID/NAME : 1509   MAGELLAN
     SERVICE DATE  : MM/DD/CCYY-MM/DD/CCYY        CLAIM TOTAL:        $8,400.00
     TRACE NUMBER  : 3JRDYQ-619999                  CLAIM ID: 38939999
     BILL TYPE     : 111              MEDICAL RECORD NUMBER: 619999
     CATEGORY CODE : A3 =REJECTED
     STS                          ERROR MESSAGE
     ---                          -------------
     21 INPATIENT CLAIMS MUST CONTAIN BOTH ACCOM AND ANCILLARY CHARGES (LOOP2400)
     ------------------------------------------------------------------------
     SUBSCR NAME:  PAUL JOHNSON
     PATIENT NAME: POLLY JOHNSON
     PAYER ID/NAME : 1509   MAGELLAN
     SERVICE DATE  : MM/DD/CCYY-MM/DD/CCYY        CLAIM TOTAL:        $9,600.00
     TRACE NUMBER  : 3JRDYR-619999                  CLAIM ID: 38939999
     BILL TYPE     : 111              MEDICAL RECORD NUMBER: 619999
     CATEGORY CODE : A3 =REJECTED
     STS                          ERROR MESSAGE
     ---                          -------------
     21 INPATIENT CLAIMS MUST CONTAIN BOTH ACCOM AND ANCILLARY CHARGES (LOOP2400)
     ------------------------------------------------------------------------
     CLAIMS ACCEPTED:       166                  AMOUNT:      258,485.76
     CLAIMS REJECTED:         2                  AMOUNT:       18,000.00
```

Summary

- Electronic media claims are submitted to insurance carriers via modem.
- Certain data (from patients, EDI receivers, insurance carriers, providers, and referring providers) has to be in place before claims can be submitted electronically.
- Electronic funds transfer can be used to submit claims by transferring funds from one bank to another.
- An electronic remittance advice explains the insurance company's response to the medical office that submitted the claim.

Review Exercises

Define the Following Terms:

1. Clearinghouse
2. Electronic media claim
3. Electronic remittance advice
4. Electronic funds transfer

Critical Thinking

Explain the advantages and disadvantages of using electronic claim management versus paper billing.

CHAPTER EIGHT

PRINTING REPORTS

■X Chapter Outline

- Introduction
- Day Sheets
  - Patient Day Sheets
  - Procedure Day Sheets
  - Payment Day Sheets
- Billing/Payment Status Report
- Analysis Reports
  - Practice Analysis Reports
  - Insurance Analysis Reports
- Aging Reports
  - Patient Aging Reports
  - Insurance Aging Reports
- Data Audit Report
- Patient Ledger
- Patient Statements
- Remainder Statements
- Custom Reports
- Summary
- Review Exercises

■X Learning Objectives

Upon completion of this chapter, the student will be able to:

- Generate various kinds of reports whose structure is provided by MediSoft.
- Use a filter to select records to display in the reports.
- Use day sheets, aging reports, patient statements, patient ledger, analysis reports, and several other reports.
- Appreciate the different uses of the many reports provided.

■X Key Terms

Billing/Payment Status Report	Insurance Aging Report	Patient Ledger
Data Audit Report	Insurance Analysis Report	Remainder Statement
Filter	Patient Day Sheet	Walkout Receipt

Introduction

MediSoft provides structures for all types of reports. The user selects the report structure and **filters** out records that he or she is not interested in by filling out a data selection screen specifying a range of chart numbers and dates. MediSoft then fills in the contents of the report, inserting data from a file into the report structure chosen.

Day Sheets

Patient Day Sheets

MediSoft provides various reports that can present data in an attractive and useful format. A patient day sheet lists the day's transactions and is used for daily reconciliation. To create a patient day sheet for Tonya Brown, click on the Reports tab, from the fly-out menu select Day Sheets then Patient Day Sheet. On the data selection screen, enter Tonya's chart number in both the From and To boxes. In the Date Created Range, change the date to read from 1/1/1900 to the present date.

Leave the Dates From Range as is. Check Show Accounts Receivable Totals and click Preview Report. Once the Preview Report button has been selected, the Day Sheet on Tonya Brown should be generated (see page 2 on the report):

Report Preview - Patient Day Sheet

100%   2 / 3   powered by crystal

Happy Valley Medical Clinic
Patient Day Sheet
September 15, 2008
ALL

Entry	Date	Document	POS	Description	Provider	Code	Modifiers	Amount
BROTO000 Brown, Tonya								
101	8/15/2008	0808110000	11	X-Ray, Chest, 2 Views	MM	71020		53.00
102	8/15/2008	0808110000	11	Check	MM	AP		-42.40
103	8/15/2008	0808110000	11	Check	MM	BP		-8.48

Patient's Charges	Patient's Receipts	Insurance Receipts	Adjustments	Patient Balance
$53.00	$0.00	-$50.88	$0.00	$2.12

Procedure Day Sheets

A patient day sheet lists procedures, codes, and amounts owed under each patient. On the other hand, a procedure day sheet lists a procedure and grouped by each separate procedure performed, the charge for each service, and a list of patient names. To create a procedure day sheet choose Reports, Day Sheets, Procedure Day Sheet. To view all procedures, leave the procedure code field blank. In the Date Created Range, change the date to read from 1/1/1900 to the present date. Leave the Dates From Range as is. Check Show Accounts Receivable and then click Preview Report. You will get a report listing every day, every patient, grouped under the procedure name (see page 2 on the report for the patient information).

Report Preview - Procedure Day Sheet

100%   2 / 5+   powered by crystal

Happy Valley Medical Clinic
Procedure Day Sheet
ALL

?_SMC_ReportTitle (String)

Entry	Date	Chart	Name	Document	POS	Debits	Credits
29130		App. of Finger Splint, Static					
96	7/14/2008	GREJE000	Green, Jenna	0808060000	11	$30.00	
		Total of 29130		Quantity: 1		$30.00	$0.00
36215		Lab Drawing Fee					
89	2/9/2006	BORJO000	Bordon, John	0602090000	11	$8.00	
		Total of 36215		Quantity: 1		$8.00	$0.00
43220		Esophageal Endoscopy					
1	12/3/2002	SIMTA000	Simpson, Tanus J	0212030000	11	$275.00	
64	4/4/2002	JONSU000	Jones, Suzy Q	0204040000	11	$275.00	
		Total of 43220		Quantity: 2		$550.00	$0.00
70373		X-Ray, Laryngography					
39	6/1/2002	WAGJE000	Wagnew, Jeremy	0206010000	11	$45.00	
		Total of 70373		Quantity: 1		$45.00	$0.00

Payment Day Sheets

Follow the same steps to generate a payment day sheet, which groups patients by their health-care providers, so the user of this report can see the payments received by each provider.

Billing/Payment Status Report

When using MediSoft Advanced version 14, you can print a billing/payment status report, which shows current billing, payment, and claim status of each transaction. To obtain this report, pull down the Reports menu and select Analysis Reports.

From the fly-out menu, select Billing/ Payment status. On the data selection screen, leave all the boxes blank. Check Show All Transactions and Preview Report. The following report is generated (see page 2 on the report for details).

Report Preview - Billing Payment Status

100%   2 / 2+

powered by crystal

Happy Valley Medical Clinic
Billing Payment Status
All Dates

?_SMC_ReportTitle (String)

Date	Document	Procedure	Amount	Policy 1	Policy 2	Policy 3	Guarantor	Adjustments	Balance
AG ADW000	**Dwight Again**	**434-5777**							
Case 2		1: Medicare (800)999-9999							
9/3/2002	0209030000	73130	45.00	12/6/2002	0.00*	0.00*	Not Billed	0.00*	45.00
9/3/2002	0209030000	99213	60.00	12/6/2002	0.00*	0.00*	Not Billed	0.00*	60.00
								Subtotal:	105.00
						Unapplied Payments and Adjustments:			0.00
								Case Balance:	105.00
Case 17		1: Medicare (800)999-9999							
		2: Aetna (602)333-3333							
11/21/2002	0211210000	99213	60.00	-72.65*	12/4/2002	0.00*	Not Billed	0.00*	-12.65
11/21/2002	0211210000	72052	80.00	-63.00*	12/4/2002	0.00*	Not Billed	0.00*	17.00
11/21/2002	0211210000	97010	10.00	-8.00*	12/4/2002	0.00*	Not Billed	0.00*	2.00
3/9/2007	0703090000	99213	60.00	Not Billed	elay Billing	0.00*	Not Billed	0.00*	60.00
								Subtotal:	66.35

Analysis Reports

Practice Analysis Reports

A practice analysis report provides a summary of activity for the period chosen and is generated usually monthly. However, it can be used for any specified time, for example, a quarter or a year. Go to Reports, click on Analysis Reports, then Practice Analysis. Leave all fields on the data selection screen blank and click Preview Report. The following report is generated:

Report Preview - Practice Analysis

100%   2 / 2+

powered by crystal

Happy Valley Medical Clinic
Practice Analysis
From 1/1/1900 to 12/31/2050

Code	Modifiers	Description	Amount	Units	Average	Costs	Net
29130		App. of Finger Splint, Static	30.00	1	30.00	5.00	25.00
36215		Lab Drawing Fee	8.00	1	8.00	3.00	5.00
43220		Esophageal Endoscopy	550.00	2	275.00	0.00	550.00
70373		X-Ray, Laryngography	45.00	1	45.00	0.00	45.00
71020		X-Ray, Chest, 2 Views	159.00	3	53.00	0.00	159.00
71030		X-Ray, Chest, Min 4 Views	65.00	1	65.00	0.00	65.00
71040		Contrast X-Ray of Bronchitis	50.00	1	50.00	0.00	50.00
72052		X-Ray, Spinal, Complete	80.00	1	80.00	0.00	80.00
73130		X-Ray, Hand, Min 3 Views	45.00	1	45.00	0.00	45.00
73562		X-Ray, Knee, Mn 3 Views	45.00	1	45.00	0.00	45.00
73610		X-Ray, Ankle, Complete	55.00	1	55.00	0.00	55.00
74283		Barium Enema, Therapeutic	110.00	1	110.00	0.00	110.00
81000		Urinalysis, Routine	22.00	2	11.00	4.00	14.00
82947		Blood Sugar Lab Test	25.00	1	25.00	12.00	13.00

As you can see, all procedure codes and descriptions are listed with the individual charges, the number of times the procedure was performed, the average charge, any costs, and the net.

Insurance Analysis Reports

An insurance analysis report can be created when using MediSoft Advanced. This report is created by pulling down the Reports menu, selecting Analysis Reports, then Insurance Analysis Report. Leave all data selection fields blank and click Preview Report.

This report lists each insurance carrier that has been billed, amounts and percentages of claims, charges, and payments.

Aging Reports

Patient Aging Reports

To create a patient aging report, pull down the Reports menu, choose Aging Reports, and select Patient Aging.

Leave all data selection questions blank and click Preview Report. As with all other reports, the details of the report start on page 2.

A patient aging report lists each patient and the amount each owes to the practice by number of days: current 0–30, past due 31–60, past due 61–90, and more than 90 days. It also lists the total amount each patient owes and each patient's phone number.

Report Preview - Patient Aging

99%   2 / 2   powered by crystal

Happy Valley Medical Clinic
Patient Aging
September 15, 2008

Chart # Name	Birthdate	Current 0 - 30	Past 31 - 60	Past 61 - 90	Past 91 +	Total Balance
AGADW000 Again, Dwight	3/30/1932	0.00	0.00	0.00 Text Object	171.35	171.35
Last Pmt: -24.65 On: 9/8/2008	434-5777					
AUSAN000 Austin, Andrew	1/1/1950	-35.00	0.00	0.00	0.00	-35.00
Last Pmt: -10.00 On: 12/22/2003	767-2222			Unapplied Pmt/Adj: -35.00		
BORJO000 Bordon, John	1/20/1972	0.00	0.00	0.00	106.00	106.00
Last Pmt: 0.00 On:	(434)777-1234					
BRIJA000 Brimley, Jay	1/23/1964	-90.00	0.00	0.00	0.00	-90.00
Last Pmt: -200.00 On: 12/22/2003	(222)342-3444			Unapplied Pmt/Adj: -200.00		
BRISU000 Brimley, Susan		0.00	0.00	0.00	12.00	12.00
Last Pmt: -48.00 On: 1/16/2002	(222)342-3444					
BROTO000 Brown, Tonya	6/14/1960	0.00	2.12	0.00	0.00	2.12
Last Pmt: -8.48 On: 8/15/2008	(212)968-5874					
CATSA000 Catera, Sammy	6/17/1964	0.00	0.00	0.00	71.00	71.00
Last Pmt: 0.00 On:	227-7722					
DOEJA000 Doe, Jane S	4/28/1962	0.00	0.00	0.00	79.00	79.00
Last Pmt: 0.00 On: 12/11/2002	(480)999-9999					

Insurance Aging Reports

Also in the Report menu is an Insurance Aging Report that lists claims filed by each insurance company by days: current 0–30 from billing date, 31–60, 61–90, and more than 90 days. The following is an example of an Insurance Aging Report:

Report Preview - Primary Insurance Aging

99%   2 / 2   powered by crystal

Happy Valley Medical Clinic
Primary Insurance Aging
September 15, 2008

Date of Service Procedure	- Past - 0 to 30	- Past - 31 to 60	- Past - 61 to 90	- Past - 91 to 120	- Past - 121 +	Total Balance
Aetna (AET00)					Erik (602)333-3333 ext: 123	
SIMTA000 Tanus J. Simpson SS:						
Birthdate: 4/4/1968 Policy: GG93-GXTA			Group: 99999			
Claim: 1 Initial Billing Date: 12/3/2002 Last Billing Date: 12/3/2002						
12/3/2002 43220	$0.00	$0.00	$0.00	$0.00	$275.00	$275.00
12/3/2002 71040	$0.00	$0.00	$0.00	$0.00	$50.00	$50.00
12/3/2002 81000	$0.00	$0.00	$0.00	$0.00	$11.00	$11.00
12/3/2002 99213	$0.00	$0.00	$0.00	$0.00	$60.00	$60.00
	$0.00	$0.00	$0.00	$0.00	$396.00	$396.00
Insurance Totals:	$0.00	$0.00	$0.00	$0.00	$396.00	$396.00
Cigna (CIG00)					Bill S. Preston 234-5678	
BRIJA000 Jay Brimley SS:						
Birthdate: 1/23/1964 Policy: 98547377			Group: 12d			
Claim: 3 Initial Billing Date: 3/25/2002 Last Billing Date: 3/25/2002						
3/25/2002 99214	$0.00	$0.00	$0.00	$0.00	$65.00	$65.00
3/25/2002 97260	$0.00	$0.00	$0.00	$0.00	$30.00	$30.00

Data Audit Report

A data audit report lists any changes or deletions made in transactions.

Patient Ledger

A **patient ledger** displays the status of each patient's account, past activity, and billing history. To print all patient ledgers, pull down the Reports menu and choose Patient Ledger. Note that the balance range and dates are already filled in. Leave these alone and click Preview Report. You can print just one patient ledger by filling in a specific patients' chart number.

The following patient account ledger groups the information under each patient's chart number and shows the patient's name, date and amount of last payment, place of service, description of the payment, procedure code, provider, and amount. It also displays a total amount for each patient.

Happy Valley Medical Clinic
Patient Account Ledger
As of 1/29/2009

Entry	Date	POS	Description	Procedure	Document	Provider	Amount
AGADW000	Dwight Again				434-5777		
	Last Payment: -24.65	On: 1/29/2009					
46	9/3/2002	11		73130	0209030000	REL	45.00
47	9/3/2002	11		99213	0209030000	REL	60.00
48	12/6/2002		Carrier: MED01 was billed	COMMENT	0209030000	REL	0.00
22	11/21/2002	11		99213	0211210000	REL	60.00
23	11/21/2002	11		72052	0211210000	REL	80.00
24	11/21/2002	11		97010	0211210000	REL	10.00
25	11/21/2002		Carrier: MED01 was billed	COMMENT	0211210000	REL	0.00
26	12/4/2002		#23664	MP	0211210000	REL	-48.00
27	12/4/2002		#23664	MP	0211210000	REL	-63.00
28	12/4/2002		#23664	MP	0211210000	REL	-8.00
29	12/4/2002		Carrier: AET00 was billed	COMMENT	0211210000	REL	0.00
91	3/9/2007	11		99213	0703090000	REL	60.00
107	1/29/2009	11	Medicare Payment	MP	0901290000	REL	-24.65
	Patient Totals						171.35
BORJO000	John Bordon				(434)777-1234		
	Last Payment: 0.00						
87	2/9/2006	11		99214	0602090000	JM	65.00
88	2/9/2006	11		82947	0602090000	JM	25.00
89	2/9/2006	11		36215	0602090000	JM	8.00
90	2/9/2006	11		99000	0602090000	JM	8.00
	Patient Totals						106.00
BRISU000	Susan Brimley				(222)342-3444		
	Last Payment: -48.00	On: 1/16/2002					
36	1/16/2002	11		CIG	0201160000	MM	-48.00
34	12/5/2002	11		99213	0212050000	MM	60.00
35	12/5/2002		Carrier: CIG00 was billed	COMMENT	0212050000	MM	0.00
37	1/16/2002		Carrier: BLU00 was billed	COMMENT	0212050000	MM	0.00
	Patient Totals						12.00
BROTO000	Tonya Brown				(212)968-5874		
	Last Payment: -42.40	On: 8/15/2008					
105	8/15/2008	11		71020	0901290000	MM	53.00
106	8/15/2008	11	Check	AP	0901290000	MM	-42.40
	Patient Totals						10.60
CATSA000	Sammy Catera				227-7722		
	Last Payment: 0.00						
77	12/6/2002	11		99213	0212060000	MM	60.00
78	12/6/2002	11		81000	0212060000	MM	11.00
	Patient Totals						71.00

Patient Statements

MediSoft provides several different statement formats. Like other reports, the patient statement can be filtered by selecting a particular date range and a specific patient or patients. To print a patient statement, click Reports then Patient Statements. The following dialog box is displayed:

Next choose Patient Statement, click OK, indicate that you would like to preview the report on the screen, and click Start. The data selection dialog box filters out all patients except Tonya Brown by choosing her chart number only.

Once Tonya Brown's chart number has been selected, click OK. The following statement appears on the screen and can be printed:

Happy Valley Medical Clinic
5222 E. Baseline Rd.
Gilbert, AZ 85234
(800)333-4747

Statement Date
9/15/2008

Page
1

Tonya Brown
229 West 109th Street
New York, NY 10025

Chart Number
BROTO000

Date	Document	Description	Case Number	Amount
			Previous Balance:	0.00

Patient: Tonya Brown   Chart #: BROTO000
   Case Description: Bronchitis   Date of Last Payment: 8/15/2008   Amount: -8.48

Date	Document	Description	Case Number	Amount
8/15/2008	0808110000	X-Ray, Chest, 2 Views	24	53.00
8/15/2008	0808110000	Aetna Payment	24	-42.40
8/15/2008	0808110000	Blue Cross/Blue Shield Payment	24	-8.48

As you can see, transactions for Tonya and her last payment are listed. The position of the two addresses at the top allows you to send these statements in window envelopes.

Remainder Statements

When using MediSoft Advanced, a **remainder statement** is sent only after all insurance carriers have paid. To generate a remainder statement, pull down the Reports menu, choose Patient Statements, and choose Remainder Statement (all payments).

Open Report

Report Title
BillFlash MS1-P
BillFlash MS3-P
BillFlash MS4-P
Patient Statement (30, 60, 90)
Patient Statement (Color)
Patient Statement (Color)(30, 60, 90)
Patient Statement (W/ Charges Only)
Patient Statement
Pre Printed Statement
Remainder Statement (All Payments)
Remainder Statement (All Pmts/Deduct)
Remainder Statement (Combined Payments)
Sample Statement w/ Image
Sample Statement w/ Logo

✔ OK

✖ Cancel

Help

☐ Show File Names

Click OK then Start to preview the report on the screen. Fill in the data selection dialog box as follows for Tonya Brown's remainder statement:

Remainder Statement (All Payments): Data Selection Questions

ATTENTION: The statement you have selected will not affect statements in Statement Management or update their submission count!

NOTE: A blank field indicates no limitation, all records will be included.

Chart Number Range: BROTO000 to BROTO000

Date From Range: ___ to ___

Insurance Carrier #1 Range: ___ to ___

Statement Total Range: 0.01 to 99999

Guarantor Billing Code Range: ___ to ___

Patient Indicator Match: ___

✔ OK

✖ Cancel

Help

Click OK. The report lists the patient's procedure, the date the procedure was performed, the amounts paid by the primary and secondary insurers, and the remainder to be billed to the guarantor.

Custom Reports

MediSoft has many custom reports. Click on the Custom Report list, and the following list is displayed:

To see the rest of the custom reports, scroll down. Choose Laser CMS (Primary) W/Form. Click OK and click Start to preview on the screen. Put in only the chart number for Michael Youngblood. Leave the remaining fields in the Data Selection dialog box blank and click OK. The filled-out CMS form will appear on the screen.

1500

HEALTH INSURANCE CLAIM FORM

PICA   PICA

1. MEDICARE	MEDICAID	TRICARE CHAMPUS	CHAMPVA	GROUP HEALTH PLAN	FECA BLK LUNG	OTHER	1a. INSURED'S I.D. NUMBER (FOR PROGRAM IN ITEM 1)
(Medicare #)	(Medicaid #)	[X] (Sponsor's SSN)	(VA File #)	(SSN or ID)	(SSN)	(ID)	USAA236678

2nd

2. PATIENT'S NAME (Last Name, First Name, Middle Initial)	3. PATIENT'S BIRTH DATE MM DD YY / SEX	4. INSURED'S NAME (Last Name, First Name, Middle Initial)
YOUNGBLOOD, MICHAEL, C	07 05 1962 M [X] F	YOUNGBLOOD, MICHAEL, C

5. PATIENT'S ADDRESS (No., Street)	6. PATIENT RELATIONSHIP TO INSURED	7. INSURED'S ADDRESS (No., Street)
73982 N. 28TH AVE.	Self [X] Spouse Child Other	73982 N. 28TH AVE.

CITY	STATE	8. PATIENT STATUS	CITY	STATE
PHOENIX	AZ	Single Married [X] Other	PHOENIX	AZ

ZIP CODE	TELEPHONE (Include Area Code)		ZIP CODE	TELEPHONE (INCLUDE AREA CODE)
85044	(602)2223333	Employed Full-Time Student [X] Part-Time Student	85044	(602)2223333

9. OTHER INSURED'S NAME (Last Name, First Name, Middle Initial)	10. IS PATIENT'S CONDITION RELATED TO:	11. INSURED'S POLICY GROUP OR FECA NUMBER
		25BB

a. OTHER INSURED'S POLICY OR GROUP NUMBER	a. EMPLOYMENT? (CURRENT OR PREVIOUS) YES NO [X]	a. INSURED'S DATE OF BIRTH MM DD YY / SEX
		07 05 1962 M [X] F

b. OTHER INSURED'S DATE OF BIRTH MM DD YY / SEX M F	b. AUTO ACCIDENT? PLACE (State) YES NO [X]	b. EMPLOYER'S NAME OR SCHOOL NAME
		ARMY

c. EMPLOYER'S NAME OR SCHOOL NAME	c. OTHER ACCIDENT? YES NO	c. INSURANCE PLAN NAME OR PROGRAM NAME

d. INSURANCE PLAN NAME OR PROGRAM NAME	10d. RESERVED FOR LOCAL USE	d. IS THERE ANOTHER HEALTH BENEFIT PLAN?
		YES NO [X] If yes, return to and complete item 9 a-d.

READ BACK OF FORM BEFORE COMPLETING AND SIGNING THIS FORM.

1st idd

12. PATIENT'S OR AUTHORIZED PERSON'S SIGNATURE. I authorize the release of any medical or other information necessary to process this claim. I also request payment of government benefits either to myself or to the party who accepts assignment below.
SIGNED   DATE 12/05/02

13. INSURED'S OR AUTHORIZED PERSON'S SIGNATURE. I authorize payment of medical benefits to the undersigned physician or supplier for services described below.
SIGNED

14. DATE OF CURRENT: ILLNESS (First symptom) OR INJURY (Accident) OR PREGNANCY(LMP) MM DD YY	15. IF PATIENT HAS HAD SAME OR SIMILAR ILLNESS. GIVE FIRST DATE MM DD YY	16. DATES PATIENT UNABLE TO WORK IN CURRENT OCCUPATION MM DD YY MM DD YY
GRADUAL INJURY		FROM TO

17. NAME OF REFERRING PHYSICIAN OR OTHER SOURCE	17a.	18. HOSPITALIZATION DATES RELATED TO CURRENT SERVICES MM DD YY MM DD YY
	17b. NPI	FROM TO

19. RESERVED FOR LOCAL USE	20. OUTSIDE LAB? $CHARGES
	YES NO [X]

21. DIAGNOSIS OR NATURE OF ILLNESS OR INJURY (RELATE ITEMS 1, 2, 3 OR 4 TO ITEM 24E BY LINE)	22. MEDICAID RESUBMISSION CODE ORIGINAL REF. NO.
1. 847.2 3. 346.9	
2. 737.30 4.	23. PRIOR AUTHORIZATION NUMBER

24. A. DATE(S) OF SERVICE From MM DD YY	To MM DD YY	B. Place of Service	C. EMG	D. PROCEDURES, SERVICES, OR SUPPLIES (Explain Unusual Circumstances) CPT/HCPCS / MODIFIER	E. DIAGNOSIS POINTER	F. $ CHARGES	G. DAYS OR UNITS	H. EPSDT Family Plan	I. ID QUAL	J. RENDERING PROVIDER ID #
									1H	HEN TRI
08 22 02	08 22 02	11		99213	123	60 00	1		NPI	
									1H	HEN TRI
08 22 02	08 22 02	11		97128	123	15 00	1		NPI	
									1H	HEN TRI
08 22 02	08 22 02	11		97010	123	10 00	1		NPI	
										NPI
										NPI
										NPI

25. FEDERAL TAX I.D. NUMBER SSN EIN	26. PATIENT'S ACCOUNT NO.	27. ACCEPT ASSIGNMENT? (For govt. claims, see back)	28. TOTAL CHARGE	29. AMOUNT PAID	30. BALANCE DUE
2222222 [X]	YOUMI000 6	[X] YES NO	$ 85 00	$	85 00

31. SIGNATURE OF PHYSICIAN OR SUPPLIER INCLUDING DEGREES OR CREDENTIALS (I certify that the statements on the reverse apply to this bill and are made a part thereof.)	32. SERVICE FACILITY LOCATION INFORMATION	33. BILLING PROVIDER INFO & PH # (800)3334747
SIGNED DATE 12/05/02	a. NPI b.	WALLACE HINCKLE MD 5222 E BASELINE RD GILBERT AZ 85234
		a. NPI b. 1H HEN TRI

NUCC Instruction Manual available at www.nucc.org

PLEASE PRINT OR TYPE

To look at superbills, choose Superbill from the Report list and click OK. Then Click OK again for the Report Title of Superbill (Numbered). Select Start to preview the report on the screen. From the drop-down list, select the chart number for Dwight Again in both the From and To Chart Number Range. Leave the data selection dialog box dates as is and enter no further information. Click OK.

1001	Happy Valley Medical Clinic 5222 E. Baseline Rd. Gilbert, AZ 85234 (800)333-4747	Date: 1/29/2009

AGADW000   Again, Dwight   1/29/2009   9:15:00 AM

EXAM	FEE	PROCEDURES	FEE	LABORATORY		FEE
New Patient		Anoscopy	46600	Aerobic Culture	87070	
Problem Focused	99201	Arthrocentesis/Aspiration/Injection		Amylase	82150	
Expanded Problem, Focused	99202	Small Joint	*20600	B12	82607	
Detailed	99203	Interm Joint	*20605	CBC & Diff	85025	
Comprehensive	99204	Major Joint	*20610	CHEM 20	80019	
Comprehnsive/High Complex	99204	Audiometry	92552	Chlamydia Screen	86317	
Initial Visit/Procedure	99025	Cast Application		Cholesterol	82465	
Well Exam Infant (up to 12 mos.)	99318	Location Long Short		Digoxin	80162	
Well Exam 1 - 4 yrs.	99382	Catherization	*53670	Electrolytes	80005	
Well Exam 5 - 11 yrs.	99383	Circumcision	54150	Ferritin	82728	
Well Exam 12 - 17 yrs.	99384	Colposcopy	*57452	Folate	82746	
Well Exam 18 - 39 yrs.	99385	Colposcopy w/Biopsy	*57454	GC Screen	87070	
Well Exam 40 - 64 yrs.	99386	Cryosurgery Premalignant Lesion		Glucose	82947	
		Location(s):		Glucose 1 HR	82950	
Established Patient		Cryosurgery Warts		Glycosylated HGB (A1C)	83036	
Minimum	99211	Location(s):		HCT	85014	
Problem Focused	99212	Curettement Lesion w/Biopsy	CTF	HDL	83718	
Expanded Problem Focused	99213	Curettement Lesion w/o Biopsy		Hep BSAG	86278	
Detailed	99214	Single	*11050	Hepatitis Profile	80059	
Comprehensive/High Complex	99215	2 - 4	*11051	HGB & HCT	85014	
Well Exam Infant(up to 12 mos.)	99391	> 4	*11052	HIV	86311	
Well exam 1 - 4 yrs.	99392	Diaphram Fitting	*57170	Iron & TIBC 83540	83550	
Well Exam 5 - 11 yrs.	99393	Ear Irrigation	69210	Kidney Profile	80007	
Well Exam 12 - 17 yrs.	99394	ECG	93000	Lead	83655	
Well Exam 18 - 39 yrs.	99395	Endometrial Biopsy	*58100	Liver Profile	82977	
Well Exam 40 - 64 yrs.	99396	Exc. Lesion w/Biopsy	CTF	Mono Test	86308	
		w/o Biopsy		Pap Smear	88155	
Obstetrics		Location Size		Pregnancy Test	84703	
Total OB Care	59400	Exc. Skin Tags (1 - 15)	*11200	Prenatal Profile	80055	
Obstetrical Visit	99212	Each Additional 10	*11201	Pro Time	85610	
Injections		Fracture Treatment		PSA	84153	
Administration Sub. / IM	90782	Loc		RPR	86592	
Drug		w/Reduc w/o Reduc		Sed. Rate	85651	
Dosage		Fracture Treatment F/U	99024	Stool Culture	87045	
Allegery	95155	I & D Abscess Single/Simple	*10060	Stool O & P	87177	
Cocci Skin Test	86490	Multiple or Comp	*10061	Strep Screen	86403	
DPT	90701	I & D Pilonidal Cyst Simple	*10080	Theophylline	80198	
Haemophilus	90737	Pilonidal Cyst Complex	10081	Thyroid Profile	80091	
Influenza	90724	IV Therapy - To One Hour	90780	TSH	84443	
MMR	90707	Each Additional Hour	*90781	Urinalysis	81000	
OPV	90712	Laceration Repair		Urine Culture	87088	
Pneumovax	90732	Location Size Sim/Comp		Draw ing Fee	36415	
TB Skin Test	86585	Laryngoscopy	31505	Specimen Collection	99000	
TD	90718	Oximetry	94760			
Unlisted Immun	90749	Punch Biopsy	CTF			
		Rhythm Strip	93040			
		Treadmill	93015			
		Trigger Point or Tendon Sheath Inj.	*20550			
		Tympanometry	92567			

Diagnosis / ICD - 9

Total Estimated Charges:

I acknowledge receipt of medical services and authorize the release of any medical information necessary to process this claim for healthcare payment only.

Tax ID Number:

I ☐ do ☐ do not authorize payment to the provider

Patient Signature

Payment Amount:

A **walkout receipt** is given to the patient when she pays. It includes procedures performed and accounting codes. To print a walkout receipt, go into the MediSoft Office Hours program, select the Reports tab, then select Custom Reports list. On the list, select Walkout Receipt (All Transactions). Click OK then Start to view the report on the screen. The following report is generated:

Summary

- MediSoft provides ready-made report structures for many kinds of statements, bills, lists, and reports.
- A patient day sheet lists every patient visit for one specified day. Information includes the procedures, place of service, providers, fees, and total balances.
- A procedure day sheet lists each specific procedure and includes the names of patients and including debits and credits.
- A payment day sheet lists each provider, all procedures performed by each provider, and the fees charged.
- A billing/payment status report presents a patient's billing status.
- A practice analysis report is generated periodically and is broken down by procedure codes. It lists charges, number of times the procedure was performed, the average charge for the procedure, costs to the practice, and the net amount.
- An insurance analysis report lists insurance carriers the practice represents, the dollar amount of outstanding claims, percent covered, charges, and payments. Each insurance carrier is listed as a primary, secondary, or tertiary.
- Patient aging reports list amounts due from patients and the number of days outstanding.
- Insurance aging reports list amounts due on claims and the number of days overdue.
- A data audit report lists any changes in transactions or appointments.
- A patient ledger lists a patient's chart number, name, the amount and date of the latest payment, provider, procedure code, and amount, as well as summary totals for each patient.
- A patient statement lists a patient's procedures, cases, and all payments received, including a balance.
- A remainder statement is a bill to the patient or guarantor after all insurance is exhausted.
- CMS-1500 is one of the many custom reports. Information from the patient's account can be printed directly onto the CMS form. Superbills and walkout receipts are also custom reports.

Review Exercises

Hands-on Exercises

1. Create a patient statement (30, 60, 90) for Michael Youngblood. Pull down the Reports menu, and choose Patient Statement (30, 60, 90). Click Start. Fill in Michael Youngblood's chart number as From and To. Click OK. Print the statement.

2. Create a patient aging statement for Michael Youngblood. Print the statement.

Matching Questions

Match the definition with the term.

_____ Patient Aging Report

_____ Remainder Statement

_____ Billing/Payment Status Report

_____ Patient Day Sheet

_____ Data Audit Report

a. report that indicates any changes and/or deletions made in the database

b. report that lists the amounts owed by a patient by how many days late the payment is

c. report that shows the status of all transactions that have a responsible carrier, showing who has paid and who has not been billed

d. report listing the day's transactions that is used for daily reconciliation

e. report that includes only procedures for which payment has been received or rejected by all applicable insurance carriers. The guarantor is responsible for the remainder.

CHAPTER NINE

DESIGNING REPORTS

Chapter Outline

- Designing Reports
- Creating a List
- Creating a Labels Report
- Creating a Custom Ledger Report
- Summary
- Review Exercises

Learning Objectives

Upon completion of this chapter, the student will:

- Be aware of the many custom bills and reports MediSoft allows the user to design.
- Know how to use the custom design grid to design several types of reports.

Key Terms

Custom Report Grid	Detail Line	Ledger
Data Fields	Footer	Report Designer
Detail	Header	Report Designer Grid

Designing Reports

With MediSoft, if your practice requires a specialized report, you can design your own modified reports, such as superbills, to meet annual code changes. MediSoft provides a grid on which you may design the structure of a report. The user indicates which table to take the data from as well as its placement. We will use two data types: text, which does not change in the report (a report header is a report header), and data fields, whose contents do change from **detail line** to detail line (because the report takes the actual data from a table that is already entered).

To design a simple report listing patient, chart number, and provider in list form, do the following:

• Click on Reports, Design Custom Reports, and Bills. You will see MediSoft's **Report Designer** with its own toolbar.

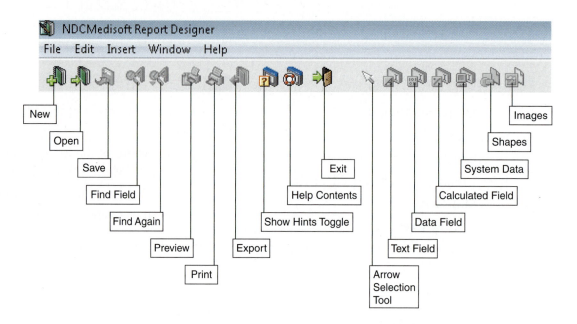

Creating a List

To create a report in list style, do the following:

• Click on the Reports tab then Design Custom Reports and Bills.
• Pull down the File menu and choose New Report. The following dialog box opens:

- Select List and click Next. The following window is displayed:

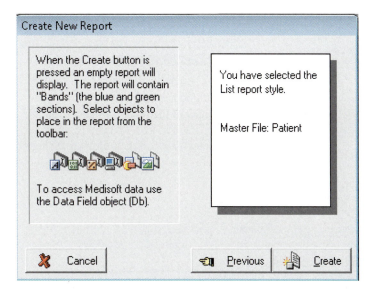

- Choose Patient as the master file and click Next.

- Click Create and the following screen, called the **Report Designer Grid**, appears. On the grid the user indicates static text fields, what fields data should be taken from, where the fields should be placed on the report, and the format of the text. All changes to the design are made on this grid.

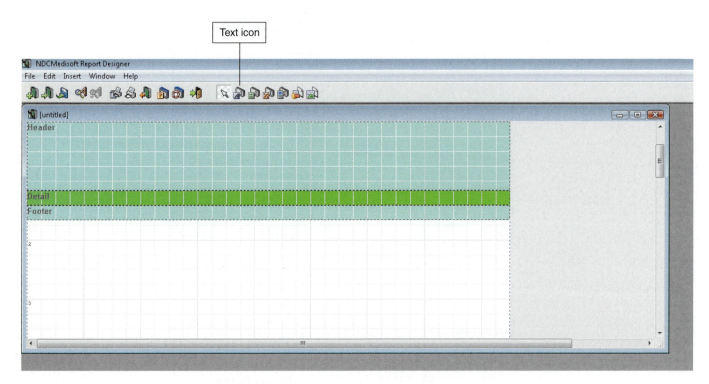

- Click on the Text Field icon on the toolbar.
- Click in the **header** area of the report designer grid, and a text box will appear on the grid. Headers are text.
- Double-click on this text box and the following dialog box will appear:

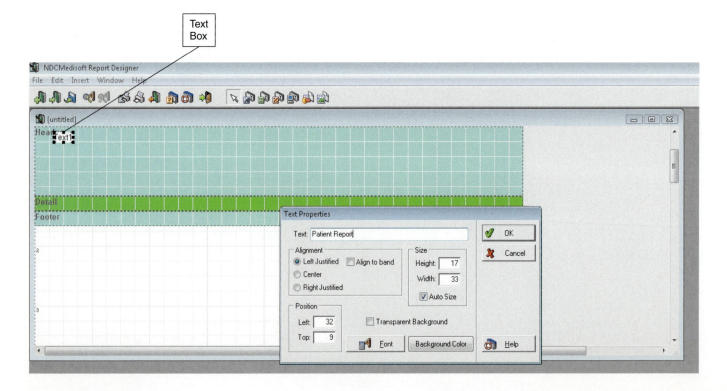

- Enter the title *(Patient Report)* and click OK.

To add detail lines (the lines of actual data), which will appear many times in the report do the following:

- Click on the Data Field icon then on the detail area of the grid. A data field box appears on the report on the detail line.

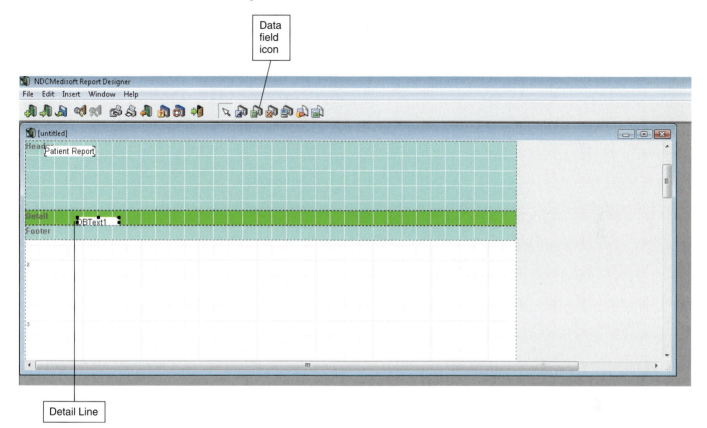

- Double-click on the Detail Data Field box, and the following dialog box will be displayed:

- When a data field is chosen, you must click New Data Field in the above dialog box. The following list of files and fields is displayed:

- You can see that it displays file names and field names from your database. First choose the file (patients); next choose a field to appear in the report. The contents of the field will be displayed in the finished report.
- Scroll down until you see Full Name (LFM). Double-click on it, and the Data Field Properties dialog box appears.

- Be sure under the Alignment option, Left Justified is selected.
- Click OK.
- Repeat this process to select the next field (Chart Number). Remember to double-click on the Data Field box and click New Data Field in the next dialog box. Choose Chart Number from the list and click OK.

On your own, add assigned provider as a data field in the detail area. Add column headers in the header area for Name (click on Text field, click on header where you want the header, double-click the text box, fill in the text with Name, and click OK), Chart Number (text), and Assigned Provider (text). In addition, add a third data field (click on the data field icon, click in the detail area where you want the field, double-click the box on the grid, click New Data Field, select the field Provider from the list of fields, then click OK). Save your changes to this report by selecting File, Save As, then typing in Patient Report and today's date. Click OK.

Add a **footer** by clicking on the text icon then clicking in the footer area. When the text box appears, double-click on it. In the Text Properties dialog box, enter Created by [Your Name]. To change the font to 9 point, click on the Font button and select 9 as the size. Click OK and click OK again.

You can change the size and style of the text by right-clicking on the text and choosing Properties. For each column header, choose bold as the style and 12 as the font size. Click OK and click OK again. Each title needs to be done separately. The report title (Patient Report) should be bold and 14 point.

Patient Report_September 26			
Patient Report			
Name	**Chart Number**	**Assigned Provider**	
Full Name	Chart	Assigned	
Created by Your Name			

Save your changes by going to File and selecting Save.

To review the report, click on the Preview Report icon. The report you designed should resemble this:

Preview Report		
1 of 1 Close Goto Page: 1		
Patient Report		
Name	**Chart Number**	**Assigned Provider**
Again,	AGADW00	REL
Austin,	AUSAN000	JM
Bordon,	BORJO000	JM
Brimley,	BRIEL000	MM
Brimley,	BRIJA000	MM
Brimley,	BRISU000	MM
Brown,	BROTO000	MM
Catera,	CATSA000	MM
Clinger,	CLIWA000	
Doe, Jane	DOEJA000	JM
Doe, John	DOEJO000	
Doogan,	DOOJA000	
Gooding,	GOOCH000	

You may not see the footer on the screen; however, if you scroll down, you will see it at the bottom. Print the report.

If you do not like the appearance of the report, for example, if headers look out of line, you can move any object around by closing the preview window and clicking on the object (e.g., text box) and dragging it around on the **custom report grid**. Its formatting can be changed by pointing to the object, right-clicking, and choosing Properties.

Creating a Labels Report

To create a labels report, pull down the File menu and choose New Report. Choose Label.

Create New Report

Reports have been categorized into several "styles". Each style defines basic report characteristics. Select the report style that matches the type of report you would like to create.

A new report can also be created from an existing report by loading the report, then saving it under a new name (use the Save As from the File menu).

Select the Report Style

- ○ List
- ● Label
- ○ Walkout Receipt
- ○ Insurance Form
- ○ Statement
- ○ Superbill
- ○ UB Insurance Form

Cancel   **Previous**   **Next**

Click Next.
In the next dialog box, select Address as the file from which to take data. Click Next.

Create New Report

Select a "Master" data file from this list to base this report from.

Only the data in this file and the files "linked" to it will be available when designing the report.

Select Master File:

- Address
- Allowed Amounts
- Appointment
- Billing Code
- Case
- Claim
- Claim Rejection Codes
- Contact
- Credit Card
- Deposit
- Diagnosis
- Electronic Claim Receiver
- Insurance Carrier
- MultiLink

Cancel   **Previous**   **Next**

In the dialog box that opens, choose Three Columns Across.

Create New Report

Select the number of columns across for your labels.

Next, measure the height of your labels (in inches).

The number of columns and label height can also be adjusted in the Report Properties window (on the File menu). To adjust the label height, select the detail band (Band 2), then make your adjustment to the band.

Columns: 3

Label Height: 1.00 Inches

Cancel   **Previous**   **Next**

Click Next. On the next screen click Create.

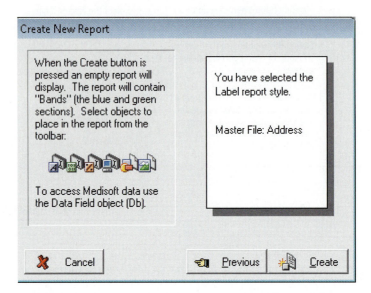

On the grid that is displayed, you are going to add data fields for the following:

Name

Street

City State ZIP

For each data field, click on the Data Field icon on the toolbar; then click in the detail line where you want it to appear. Double-click the Data Field box, click New Field, choose the field from the list, and click OK. If you want to, try to add a comma between city and state—it is a text field. Save the report as Mailing Labels.

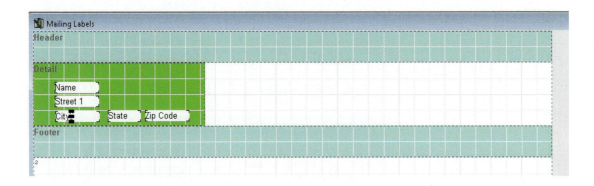

Preview the report. If you do not like the way it looks, close the preview screen and move the field names around on the grid until you like the appearance.

Creating a Custom Ledger Report

When using MediSoft Advanced, a report in ledger style can be created. To create a report in **ledger** style, pull down the Reports menu and select Design Custom Reports and Bills. Click the New icon on the report designer toolbar.

Select Ledger and click Next. In the dialog box that opens, select Patient as the master file.

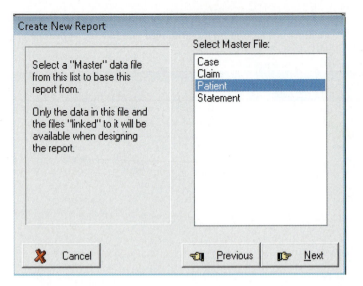

Click Next.
In the next dialog box that opens, select Case as the detail file.

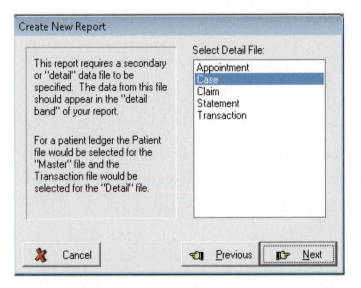

Click Next.
The following window should be displayed:

Click Create and the following screen should be displayed:

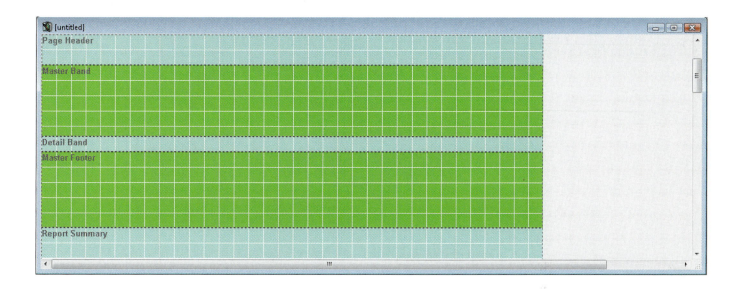

Click on the Data Field icon on the toolbar and click in the Master Band section of the screen. A text box will appear. Double-click on the box, and the following window opens:

Click the New Data Field button. Select Patient as the file.

Choose Patient Full Name (LFM) as the data field. Click OK. In the Data Field Properties window, click OK.

To add detail lines, click on the Data Field icon; then click in the detail band. Double-click on the text box that opens. Choose Case as the file and Diagnosis 1 as the data field.

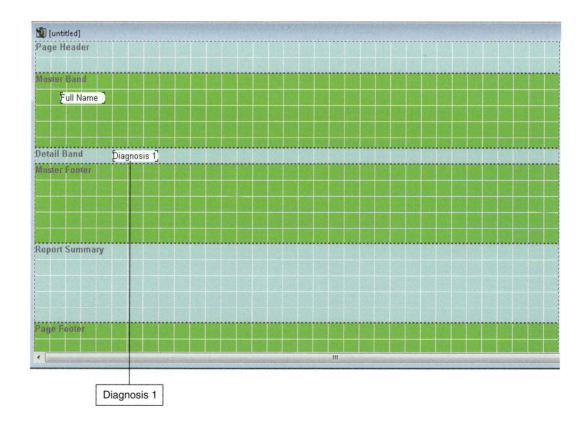

Click OK then OK again. The Diagnosis 1 field should now be seen on the report:

Print Patient Statements can also be added as a data field in the detail band. This is done in the same way as we just used for adding the Diagnosis 1 field in the detail band.

Using the text field, a page footer with the name of the individual who has created the report can be added.

A report title can be added as a page header in the same manner.

The font size for the report title can be changed by double-clicking on the title, clicking on Font, and changing the size to 16 point and the style to bold.

For this report, in the Master Band area, the following information is added (both text fields): Diagnosis (bold, 12 point) and Patient Statement Printed (bold, 12 point).

Save the report as Diagnosis Report and click OK.

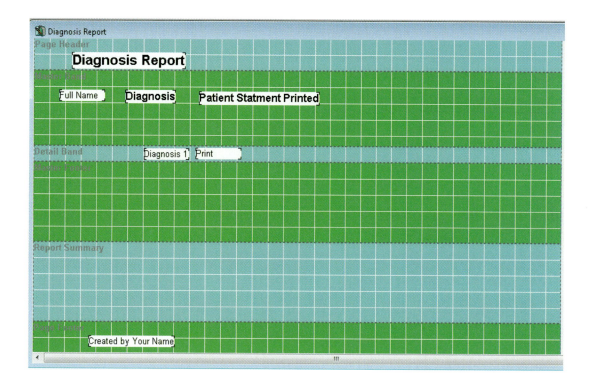

Click the Preview icon. The report should resemble the following:

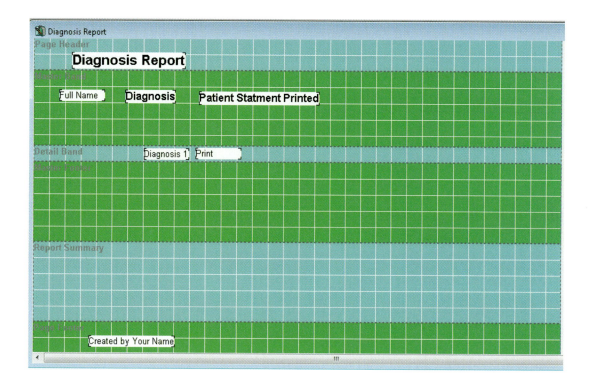

Print the report.

Summary

- MediSoft allows the user to design custom reports and statements.
- The user may choose the style from a dialog box: list, label, ledger, walkout receipt, insurance form, or statement.
- The user employs the custom design grid to arrange and format text and fields from one or more tables.

Review Exercises

Define the Following Terms:

data field

detail line

footer

header

Identify the Buttons on the Report Designer Toolbar by Filling in the Empty Boxes:

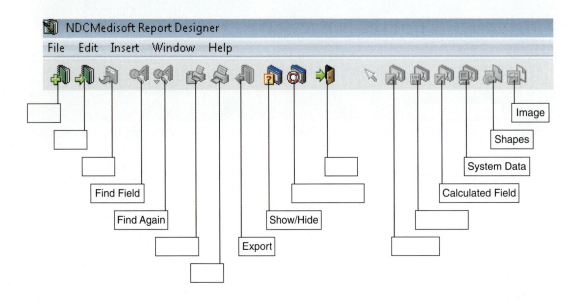

Find Field

Find Again

Export

Show/Hide

Calculated Field

System Data

Shapes

Image

CHAPTER TEN

SETTING UP A NEW PRACTICE

Chapter Outline

- HIPAA Compliance
- Entering Practice Information
- Entering Provider Information
- Entering Address Information
- Entering Patient Information
- Entering Insurance Carriers
- Entering Diagnosis Codes
- Entering Procedure, Payment, and Adjustment Codes
- Entering Cases
- Transaction Entry and Claim Management
- Printing Reports
- Summary

Learning Objectives

Upon completion of this chapter, the student will be able to establish a new practice database using MediSoft, including the following:

- Making the practice HIPAA compliant
- Entering practice information
- Entering provider information
- Entering address information
- Entering patient information
- Entering insurance carriers
- Entering diagnoses codes
- Entering billing codes
- Entering procedure, payment, and adjustment codes
- Entering and editing patient profiles and cases
- Entering transactions and creating claims
- Generating reports
- Viewing the deposit list

HIPAA Compliance

MediSoft version 14 allows you to choose options that allow your program to comply with the Health Insurance Portability and Accountability Act of 1996 (HIPAA), which set privacy standards for patient information. For the purpose of this text, do *not* turn the auto log off. Once a user is logged off, he will need a password to log back into the program; this helps guard against unauthorized use of the program and protects privacy. If you perform the following steps using the MediSoft demo, you will not be able to log back in, virtually making your MediSoft program unworkable.

In a medical office, to turn it off, you would pull down the File menu, choose Program Options, click on the HIPAA tab, click on Auto Log Off and Warn on Unapproved Codes. Then click the Save button.

Entering Practice Information

If you are starting a new practice or computerizing an existing practice using MediSoft, there are several tasks you need to complete. To set up a new database file, do the following:

• Pull down the File menu and choose New Practice.

The following dialog box will be displayed:

Create a new set of data

Enter the practice or doctor's name to identify this set of data:

_____

Enter the data path:

C:\MediData\ _____ | Browse

✔ Create
✘ Cancel
Help

- Enter the practice name *(Dr. Phiyllis Malloy).* You need to create a folder for the database.
- Your data path will be C:\MediData\Malloy so enter *Malloy* in the Enter the Data Path text box.

Create a new set of data

Enter the practice or doctor's name to identify this set of data:

Dr Phiyllis Malloy

Enter the data path:

C:\MediData\ Malloy | Browse

✔ Create
✘ Cancel
Help

- Click Create.
- In the confirm dialog box that opens, click Yes.

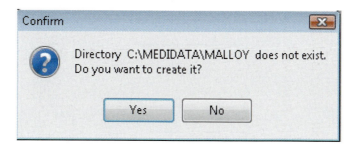

Confirm

❓ Directory C:\MEDIDATA\MALLOY does not exist.
Do you want to create it?

Yes   No

The following dialog box will be displayed:

Practice Information

Practice | Billing Service

Practice Name:	
Street:	
City:	State:
Zip Code:	
Phone:	Extension:
Fax Phone:	
Type:	▼
Federal Tax ID:	
Extra 1:	
Extra 2:	
Entity Type:	▼

Save
Cancel
Help

- Fill in Dr. Malloy's practice information as presented below and Save the record.

Practice Information

Practice | Billing Service

Practice Name:	Dr. Phiyllis Malloy
Street:	125 West 100th Street
City:	New York	State: NY
Zip Code:	10025
Phone:	(212)555-5555	Extension: 444
Fax Phone:	(212)555-5556
Type:	Medical ▼
Federal Tax ID:	000000000
Extra 1:	
Extra 2:	
Entity Type:	▼

Save
Cancel
Help

Entering Provider Information

Next you need to enter provider information for Dr. Malloy. To enter provider information, do the following:

- Pull down the Lists menu, click Provider, and select Providers in the fly-out menu, or simply click on the Provider icon.
- On the Provider List window, click New.
- Add the following information:

Provider: Malloy, Phiyllis

| Address | Default Pins | Default Group IDs | PINs | Eligibility |

Code: [ ]   If the Code is left blank, the program will assign one.   ☐ Inactive

Save

Cancel

Help

Last Name: Malloy   Middle Initial: [ ]
First Name: Phiyllis   Credentials: MD PHD
Street: 125 West 100th Street
[ ]
City: New York   State: NY
Zip Code: 10025
E-Mail: [ ]
Office: (212)555-5555   Fax: (212)555-5556
Home: [ ]   Cell: [ ]

☑ Signature On File   Signature Date: 9/17/2008 ▼
☑ Medicare Participating   License Number: [ ]

Specialty: General Practice ▼ 001
Entity Type: Person ▼

- Click the Save button to save your entry.
- To enter Dr. Malloy's default PIN information, click on Edit on the Provider List window.

Edit

- Click the Default PINs tab (under the toolbar), and enter the following:

- Click the Save button to save your entry. Then close the Provider List window.

Entering Address Information

The MediSoft software program provides the capability of storing address information that is important to the practice. To enter information in the address list, either click on the Address icon on the toolbar or pull down the Lists menu and choose Addresses. Click the New button. In the dialog box that opens, do not fill in the Code field; instead tab over the Code field, enter the following information, and choose the Type from the drop-down list:

Medisoft Demo - Dr Phiyllis Malloy

File Edit Activities Lists Reports Tools Window Services Help

Address List

Search for:

Code	Name

Edit   New

Address: Adams, Joan Q.

Code: [   ]   If the Code is left blank, the program will assign one.

Name: Adams, Joan Q.
Street: 540 Broadway
[   ]
City: New York   State: NY
Zip Code: 10025

Type: Miscellaneous
Phone: [   ]   Extension: [   ]
Fax Phone: [   ]
Cell Phone: [   ]
Office: [   ]
Contact: [   ]
E-Mail: [   ]
ID: [   ]
Identifier: [   ]

Entity ID: [   ]   Purchased Services: ☐
Mammography Certification: [   ]
Extra 1: [   ]   Extra 2: [   ]

Save
Cancel
Help

F1 Help   F3 Save   Esc Cancel

- Once your information has been saved, MediSoft will assign a code to the patient. The information will appear on the address list.

Code →

Code	Name	Street 1	Str
ADA00	Adams, Joan Q.	540 Broadway	

Address List

Search for: Field: Type

Edit   New   Delete   Close

- Perform the same steps to enter the rest of the patients' addresses.

Add the following to the address list (each type is miscellaneous) and be sure to save your work after adding each record:

Santiago, Rose
135 East 102nd Street
New York, NY 10025

Shah, James
345 Amsterdam Avenue
New York, NY 10025

Wang, Amy
444 Central Park West
New York, NY 10025

Wang, Karen
444 Central Park West
New York, NY 10025

Williams, Franklin D.
125 Columbus Avenue
New York, NY 10025

Add a record for yourself.

Still using the Address List dialog box, now you need to create new records for the following employers. For the first employer, enter the following:

Address: Middlesex County College				
Code: [ ]	If the Code is left blank, the program will assign one.			Save
Name:	Middlesex County College			Cancel
Street:	2600 Woodbridge Avenue			Help
	[ ]			
City:	Edison	State:	NJ	
Zip Code:	08816			
Type:	Employer ▼			
Phone:	(732)555-2526	Extension: [ ]		
Fax Phone:	[ ]			
Cell Phone:	[ ]			
Office:	[ ]			
Contact:	[ ]			
E-Mail:	[ ]			
ID:	[ ]			
Identifier:	[ ]			
Entity ID: [ ]	Purchased Services: ☐			
	Mammography Certification: [ ]			
Extra 1: [ ]	Extra 2: [ ]			

Once the record has been saved, a Code will be assigned:

	Code	Name	Street 1	Street 2	City
▶	ADA00	Adams, Joan Q	540 Broadway		New York
	MID00	Middlesex County College	2600 Woodbridge Avenue		Edison
	SAN00	Santiago, Rose	135 East 102nd Street		New York
	SHA00	Shah, James	345 Amsterdam Avenue		New York
	WAN0	Wang, Amy	444 Central Park West		New York
	WAN0	Wang, Karen	444 Central Park West		New York
	WIL00	Willaims, Franklin D.	125 Columbus Avenue		New York

Code

Enter a second employer:

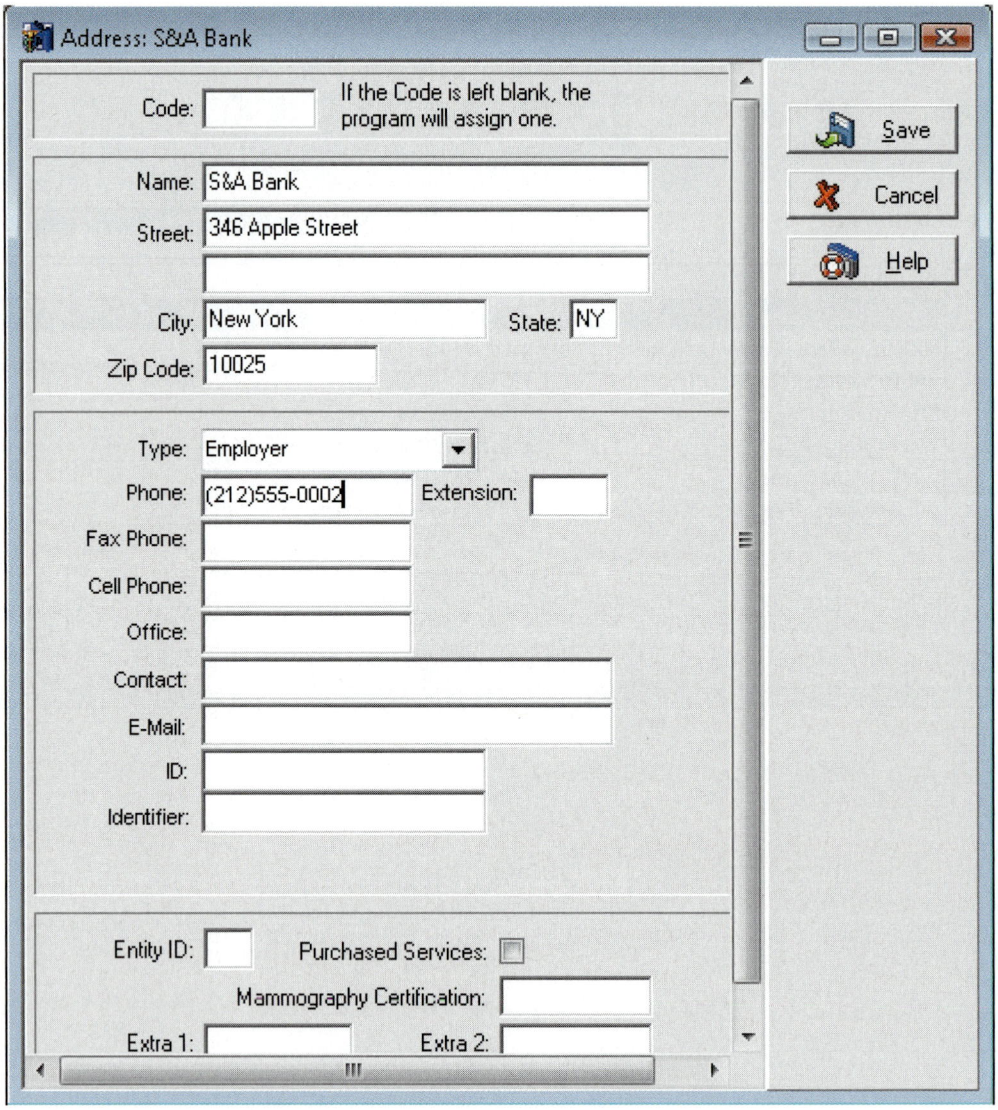

Add a third employer:

Address: Micro-Mania			

Code: [   ]   If the Code is left blank, the program will assign one.

Name: [Micro-Mania]

Street: [247 West 125th Street]

[   ]

City: [New York]   State: [NY]

Zip Code: [10025]

Type: [Employer ▼]

Phone: [   ]   Extension: [   ]

Fax Phone: [   ]

Cell Phone: [   ]

Office: [   ]

Contact: [   ]

E-Mail: [   ]

ID: [   ]

Identifier: [   ]

Entity ID: [   ]   Purchased Services: [ ]

Mammography Certification: [   ]

Extra 1: [   ]   Extra 2: [   ]

Save

Cancel

Help

After saving this information, check to see if the Field box on the Address List indicates that the list will be sorted by Code. Be sure and select Code from the drop-down field list. By selecting Code, all of your entries will be organized alphabetically by code. With the Code selected, your address list should resemble this:

If in the Field box, Type is selected, your employer entries will be seen first in the address list window, with patient entries following.

Entering Patient Information

You need to enter a list of patients that use Dr. Malloy's practice. Do the following:

- To enter patient data, click on the Patient List icon and select the New button or pull down the Lists menu and choose Patients/Guarantors and Cases.
- Click New.
- Enter the following information in the name and address page of the dialog box:
  - Last Name   Adams
  - First Name   Joan
  - Middle Initial   Q
  - Street   540 Broadway
  - ZIP   10025
  - City   New York
  - State   NY
  - Phone   2125559999
  - Birth Date   5/25/1946
  - Sex   Female
  - SSN   111111111
- However, do not enter a chart number. MediSoft will automatically enter it for you when you save the record.
- Click the Other Information tab, and enter the employer (MID00), employment status (part time). Check signature on file and enter 5/10/1979 as the date. This means she will not have to sign each insurance form.
- Save the record.
- You will be brought back to the Patient List.

- Click New to add a new patient.
- Enter the following information in the name and address page of the dialog box:
  - Last Name   Williams
  - First Name   Franklin
  - Middle Initial   D
  - Street   125 Columbus Avenue
  - ZIP   10025
  - City   New York
  - State   NY
  - Phone   2125557777
  - Birth Date   2/7/1953
  - Sex   Male
  - SSN   333333333
- Click the Other Information tab, and enter the assigned provider (PM). His employer is Micro-Mania, and he is employed full time. Check signature on file and enter 2/10/1995 as the date.
- Save the record, and MediSoft assigns a chart number.

- Click New to add a third patient:
- Enter the following information in the name and address page of the dialog box:
  - Last Name   Shah
  - First Name   James
  - Middle Initial
  - Street   343 Amsterdam Avenue
  - ZIP   10025
  - City   New York
  - State   NY
  - Phone   2125552222
  - Birth Date   7/14/1960

- Sex   Male
- SSN   222222222
- Click the Other Information tab, and enter the assigned provider (PM). His employer is S&A Bank; he is employed full time. Check signature on file and enter 2/10/1985 as the date.
- Save the record and MediSoft assigns a chart number.

- Click New to add another patient.
- Enter the following information on the name and address page of the dialog box:
    - Last Name   Cohen
    - First Name   Miriam
    - Middle Initial   B
    - Street   785 West End Avenue
    - ZIP   10025
    - City   New York
    - State   NY
    - Phone   2125556710
    - Birth Date   5/7/1937
    - Sex   Female
    - SSN   555555555
- Click the Other Information tab, and enter the assigned provider (PM). Check signature on file and enter 5/10/1955 as the date.
- Save the record and MediSoft assigns a chart number.

- Click New.
- Enter the following information in the name and address page of the dialog box:
    - Last Name   Santiago
    - First Name   Rosa
    - Middle Initial
    - Street   135 East 102 Street
    - ZIP   10025
    - City   New York
    - State   NY
    - Phone   2125558888
    - Birth Date   9/6/1973
    - Sex   Female
    - SSN   444444444
- Click the Other Information tab, and enter the assigned provider (PM).
- Save the record.

- Click New (before entering each patient's record).
- Enter the following information in the name and address page of the dialog box.
    - Last Name   Wang
    - First Name   Amy
    - Middle Initial
    - Street   444 Central Park West
    - ZIP   10025
    - City   New York
    - State   NY
    - Phone   2125550000
    - Birth Date   7/25/2001
    - Sex   Female
    - SSN   666666666
- Click the Other Information tab, and enter the assigned provider (PM).
- Save the record.

- Click New.
- Enter the following information in the name and address page of the dialog box.
  - Last Name   Wang
  - First Name   Karen
  - Middle Initial
  - Street   444 Central Park West
  - ZIP   10025
  - City   New York
  - State   NY
  - Phone   2125550000
  - Birth Date   5/3/1970
  - Sex   Female
  - SSN   777777777
- Click the Other Information tab, and enter the assigned provider (PM). Check signature on file and enter 3/30/1995 as the date.
- Save the record.

- Click New and add a record for yourself as a patient. Include your real name. Your provider is Dr. Malloy. You can make up the rest of the information. Save the record.

The patient list should resemble the following with the additional record for yourself:

Note that Joan Q. Adams has no provider assigned. Edit her record by double-clicking on her name and clicking the Other Information tab. Enter PM as her provider; then save the record.

Each time a new patient is entered, MediSoft assigns a chart number. If you cannot view the chart number on the Patient List, close out the Patient List then select Lists from the toolbar and go into Patient/Guarantors and Cases to view the lists where now the chart numbers will appear.

Entering Insurance Carriers

You also need to create a list of insurance carriers.

- Pull down the Lists menu and choose Insurance then Carriers.

The following dialog box opens:

- Click New.
- Add the following information:
  - Name   Aetna
  - Address   PO Box 960
  - City   Bluebell
  - State   PA
  - ZIP   19422
  - Phone   8005551122
  - Extension   4
  - Fax   8005551123
  - Contact   Jane Smith
- Click the Options tab. Click the down arrow next to Type and scroll down to select HMO.
- Save the record and MediSoft assigns a code.

- Click New.
- Add a second carrier with the following information:
  - Name   Blue Cross/Blue Shield
  - Address   88 Broad Street
  - City   Philadelphia
  - State   PA
  - ZIP   17109
  - Phone   2155559089
  - Extension   49
  - Fax   2155559088
  - Contact
- Click the Options tab. Click the down arrow next to Type and select Blue Cross/Shield.
- Save the record and MediSoft assigns a code.

- Click New.
- Add a third carrier with the following information:
  - Name   Medicaid
  - Address   123 Broadway
  - City   New York
  - State   NY
  - ZIP   10025
  - Phone   2125555675
  - Extension   49
  - Fax   2125559088
  - Contact
- Click the Options tab. Click the down arrow next to Type and select Medicaid.
- Save the record and MediSoft assigns a code.

- Click New.
- Add a carrier with the following information:
  - Name   Medicare
  - Address   89 Main Street
  - City   Newark
  - State   NJ
  - ZIP   06000
  - Phone   2735554321
  - Extension   6789
  - Fax   2735554322
  - Contact

- Click the Options tab. Click the down arrow next to Type and select Medicare.
- Save the record and MediSoft assigns a code.

- Add carriers with the following information, and remember to click New before each carrier:
  - Name   CIGNA
  - Address   123 West 73rd Street
  - City   New York
  - State   NY
  - ZIP   10025
  - Phone   2125555675
  - Extension
  - Fax   2125555678
  - Contact
- Click the Options tab. Click the down arrow next to Type and select HMO.
- Save the record and MediSoft assigns a code.

- Click New.
  - Name   Hancock Worker's Compensation
  - Address   1 Delaware Street
  - City   Washington
  - State   DC
  - ZIP   30000
  - Phone   8005551074
  - Extension
  - Fax   8005551075
  - Contact
- Click the Options tab. Click the down arrow next to Type and select Worker's Comp.
- Save the record and MediSoft assigns a code.

  Your insurance carrier list should resemble the following:

Entering Diagnosis Codes

You now need to add a list of the diagnoses common to Dr. Malloy's practice. To add a diagnoses list, do the following:

- Pull down the Lists menu and choose Diagnosis codes. Diagnosis codes are added one at a time.
- Click New and fill in the following information:
  - Code 1   034.0
  - Description   Strep Throat

- Save the record.
- Click New and fill in the following information to add another diagnosis code:
  - Code 1   052.9
  - Description   Chicken Pox
- Save the record.

On your own, add the rest of the diagnosis codes:

Code 1	Code 2	Code 3	Codes On Disk	Description
052.9	052.9	052.9	False	Chicken Pox
346.9	346.9	346.9	False	Headache-Migraine
422.9	422.9	422.9	False	Heart Disease
401.9	4019	4019	False	Hypertension
250.01	250.01	250.01	False	IDDM Diabetes Mellitis
724.2	724.2	724.2	False	Low Back Pain
075.0	075.0	075.0	False	Mononucleosis
034.0	034.0	034.0	False	Strep Throat
469.9	469.9	469.9	False	Upper Respiratory Infection

Diagnosis List — Search for: Field: Description

Edit | New | Delete | Close

Entering Procedure, Payment, and Adjustment Codes

The method in which procedure, payment, and adjustment codes are entered depends on the version of MediSoft you are using. When using MediSoft Basic, CPT codes are entered in the system as follows:

- Click on the CPT icon or pull down the Lists menu and select Procedure, Payment, and Adjustment list. Click New. A two-tabbed dialog box is displayed. You will need to fill in information on each page of the dialog box for each code.
- Enter 36215 as Code 1.
- Enter Lab Drawing Fee as the description.

- Click on Inside Lab Charge as the code type (select it using the code type drop-down list).

Medisoft Demo - Dr Phiyllis Malloy - [Procedure/Payment/Adjustment: Lab Drawing Fee]

File   Edit   Activities   Lists   Reports   Tools   Window   Services   Help

General | Amounts

Code 1: 36215   ☐ Inactive

Description: Lab Drawing Fee

Code Type: Inside lab charge ▼

Account Code: [   ]   ┌─ Alternate Codes ─┐

Type of Service: 5   2: 36215

Place of Service: [   ]   3: 36215

Time To Do Procedure: 0

Don't Bill To Insurance: [   ]

Only Bill To Insurance: [   ]

Default Modifiers: [ ][ ][ ][ ]

Revenue Code: [▼][🔍]

Default Units: 0

National Drug Code: [   ]

Code ID Qualifier: [   ]

- Enter 5 as Type of Service. The type of service is very important to indicate correctly since this identifies if the service is a charge, payment, adjustment, or procedure.
- Enter 0 as Time to Do Procedure.
- Click on the Amounts tab and enter 8 as Charge Amount A.

Medisoft Demo - Dr Phiyllis Malloy - [Procedure/Payment/Adjustment: Lab Drawing Fee]

File   Edit   Activities   Lists   Reports   Tools   Window   Services   Help

General | **Amounts**

Charge Amounts

A: 8

The amount refers to the price charged for the service by the practice.
- Save the record.

Add the rest of the information for the codes, description, amounts, and types as listed here: (Be very careful to enter the correct type for each code.)

CODE	DESCRIPTION	AMOUNT	TYPE DESCRIPTION
71020	X-ray, Chest 2 Views	$53.00	Procedure charge
80050	General Health Screen Panel	$45.00	Outside lab charge
82954	Glucose Test	$10.00	Inside lab charge
84704	Pregnancy Test	$25.00	Inside lab charge
85023	CBC	$18.00	Inside lab charge
87072	Culture, Strep Throat	$15.00	Procedure charge
93000	Electrocardiogram-Interp/Report	$45.00	Procedure charge
97010	Hot/Cold Pack Therapy	$10.00	Procedure charge
99213	Office Visit Established Patient	$225.00	Procedure charge
AP	Aetna Payment	$0.00	Insurance payment
BLU	Blue Cross/Blue Shield	$0.00	Insurance payment
BLUADJ	Blue Cross/Adjustment	$0.00	Insurance adjustment
CASH	Cash Payment – Thanks!	$0.00	Cash payment
CHECK	Personal Check Payment	$0.00	Check Payment
CIG	CIGNA Payment	$0.00	Insurance payment
CIGWROFF	CIGNA Write-off	$0.00	Insurance adjustment
COPAYCASH	Cash Copayment	$0.00	Cash copayment

An advantage of using the MediSoft Advanced version 14 is that when you enter procedure and payment codes you can enter the allowed amount that is the contracted dollar amount that the insurance company pays the practice for each service. For example, it may pay 80 percent of the allowed amount. MediSoft uses the allowed amount to calculate insurance repsonsiblity, patient responsibility, and adjustments. The 20 percent—the difference between the allowed amount and the insurance payment—is the patient's responsibility. The difference between the allowed amount and the full charge (called an adjustment) is written off by the practice.

To enter the allowed amount using MediSoft Advanced, do the following:

- Click on the CPT icon or pull down the Lists menu and select Procedure, Payment, and Adjustment List. Click New. A three-tabbed dialog box is displayed.
- Enter 97540 as Code 1.
- Enter Phys Therapy/Life Management as the description.
- Enter Procedure charge as the code type (select it using the drop-down list).

- Enter A as service classification.

Procedure/Payment/Adjustment: Phys Therapy/Life Mgmt

General | Amounts | Allowed Amounts

Code 1: **97540**   ☐ Inactive

Description: Phys Therapy/Life Mgmt

Code Type: Procedure charge ▼

Account Code: [   ]

Type of Service: [ ]   ┌─ Alternate Codes ─┐
                                2: 97540
Place of Service: [ ]   3: 97540

Time To Do Procedure: 0

Service Classification: A ▼

Don't Bill To Insurance: [   ]

Only Bill To Insurance: [   ]

Default Modifiers: [ ][ ][ ][ ]

Revenue Code: [   ] ▼ 🔍

Default Units: 0

National Drug Code: [   ]

Code ID Qualifier: [ ]

☐ Taxable   ☐ Patient Only Responsible
☐ HIPAA Approved   ☐ Purchased Service
☐ Require Co-pay
☑ HCPCS Code

UB HCPCS Code: 97540

[Save] [Cancel] [Help]

- Click on the Amounts tab and enter 30 as Charge Amount A.

Procedure/Payment/Adjustment: Phys Therapy/Life Mgmt

General | **Amounts** | Allowed Amounts

Charge Amounts

A: 30	H: 0.00	O: 0.00	V: 0.00
B: 0.00	I: 0.00	P: 0.00	W: 0.00
C: 0.00	J: 0.00	Q: 0.00	X: 0.00
D: 0.00	K: 0.00	R: 0.00	Y: 0.00
E: 0.00	L: 0.00	S: 0.00	Z: 0.00
F: 0.00	M: 0.00	T: 0.00	
G: 0.00	N: 0.00	U: 0.00	

Cost of Service/Product: 0.00   Medicare Allowed Amount: 0.00

Save
Cancel
Help

- Click on the Allowed Amounts tab, and enter the following information (save the record when you are done):

Procedure/Payment/Adjustment: Phys Therapy/Life Mgmt

General | Amounts | **Allowed Amounts**

Insurance Name	Code	Modifiers	Amount	UB Non-Covere
Aetna	AET00		15.50	☐
Blue Cross/Blue Shield	BLU00		15.50	☐
CIGNA	CIG00		15.00	☐
Hancock Worker's Compensation	HAN00		10.00	☐
Medicaid	MED00		13.45	☐
▶ Medicare	MED01		13.00	☐

Save
Cancel
Help

Unlike MediSoft Advanced, the Basic version does not allow for the entering of allowed amounts in the procedure/payment/adjustment area. Instead, allowed amounts must be added in the transaction payment area as a write-off. In MediSoft Advanced, adjustments and write-offs are also entered on this list. In MediSoft Basic, these are entered under Payments and Adjustments in the Transaction window. An adjustment is a positive or negative change in a patient's charge. For instance, a charge may be added to a patient's account if the account is sent to a collection agency. An adjustment is entered in the same way as a payment and needs to be applied to the patient's account after all insurance payments have been made.

If the above table information were entered into MediSoft Advanced, the grid containing the information would appear as follows:

NDCMedisoft Advanced - Dr Phiyllis Malloy

File Edit Activities Lists Reports Tools Window Services Help

Procedure/Payment/Adjustment List

Search for: _____   Field: Code 1

Code 1	Description	Amount	Type Description
36215	Lab Drawing Fee	$8.00	Inside lab charge
71020	X-ray, Chest 2 Views	$53.00	Procedure charge
80050	General Health Screen Panel	$45.00	Outside lab charge
82954	Glucose Test	$10.00	Inside lab charge
84704	Pregnancy Test	$25.00	Inside lab charge
85023	CBC	$18.00	Inside lab charge
87072	Culture, Strep Throat	$15.00	Procedure charge
93000	Electrocardiogram-Interp/Report	$45.00	Procedure charge
97010	Hot/Cold Pack Therapy	$10.00	Procedure charge
97540	Phys Therapy/Life Mgmt	$30.00	Procedure charge
99213	Office Visit Established Patient	$225.00	Procedure charge
AP	Aetna Payment	$0.00	Insurance payment
BLU	Blue Cross/Blue Shield	$0.00	Insurance payment
BLUEADJ	Blue Cross/Adjustment	$0.00	Insurance Adjustment
CASH	Cash Payment - Thanks	$0.00	Cash payment
CHECK	Personal Check Payment	$0.00	Check payment
CIG	CIGNA Payment	$0.00	Insurance payment
CIGWROFF	CIGNA Write-off	$0.00	Insurance Adjustment
COPAYCASH	Cash Copayment	$0.00	Cash co-payment

Edit   New   Delete   Print Grid   Close

Using MediSoft Advanced, enter an allowed amount for a general health screen by doing the following: pull down the Lists menu, choose Procedures/Payment/Adjustment, double-click on General Health Screen, and click the Allowed Amounts tab. Enter the following:

Procedure/Payment/Adjustment: General Health Screen Panel

General | Amounts | **Allowed Amounts**

Insurance Name	Code	Modifiers	Amount	UB Non-Cover
Aetna	AET00		35.00	☐
Blue Cross/Blue Shield	BLU00		35.00	☐
CIGNA	CIG00		35.00	☐
Hancock Worker's Compensation	HAN00		20.00	☐
Medicaid	MED00		30.00	☐
Medicare	MED01		20.00	☐

Save   Cancel   Help

● For a strep throat culture, add the following allowed amounts:

Insurance Name	Code	Modifiers	Amount	
Aetna	AET00		15.00	
Blue Cross/Blue Shield	BLU00		15.00	
CIGNA	CIG00		10.00	
Hancock Worker's Compensation	HAN00		5.00	
Medicaid	MED00		9.00	
Medicare	MED01		12.00	

Procedure/Payment/Adjustment: Culture, Strep Throat — Allowed Amounts tab (General | Amounts | Allowed Amounts). Buttons: Save, Cancel, Help.

Entering Cases

Using your MediSoft Demo or the Advanced version, enter a new case for Joan Q. Adams by doing the following:

● Click on the Patient List icon or pull down the Lists menu and select Patients/Guarantors and Cases.
● Click on Joan Q. Adams, and click the Case option button.
● Click the New Case.
● The Personal tab is the default tab.

Medisoft Demo – Dr Phiyllis Malloy. Menu: File, Edit, Activities, Lists, Reports, Tools, Window, Services, Help.

Patient List — Search for: Field: Chart Number. Patient / Case.

Chart Nu...	Last Name	First Name	Middle Initial	Street 1	Street 2
ADAJO000	Adams	Joan	Q	540 Broadway	
COHMI000	Cohen	Miriam	B	785 West End Avenue	
SANRO000					
SHAJA000					
WANAM000					
WANKA000					
WILFR000					

Case: ADAJO000 Adams, Joan Q (new). Tabs: Condition, Miscellaneous, Medicaid and Tricare, Comment, EDI, Personal, Account, Diagnosis, Policy 1, Policy 2, Policy 3.

Case Number: 0

Description: ☐ Cash Case
Global Coverage Until: ☑ Print Patient Statement
Guarantor: ADAJO000   Adams, Joan Q
Marital Status: Student Status:

Buttons: Save, Cancel, Help, UB04..., Eligibility...

Employment
Employer: MID00   Middlesex County College

Fill in the description, the marital status, and the student status as shown below:

The rest of the information has already been entered or provided by MediSoft.

- Click on the Account tab, click on the arrow in the Provider drop-down list, and select Dr. Malloy.

- Click on the Diagnosis tab, and select Strep Throat from the Principal Diagnosis 1 drop-down list. (The principal diagnosis represents the diagnosis for which the patient is being seen.)

Case: ADAJO000 Adams, Joan Q [Strep Throat]

| Condition | Miscellaneous | Medicaid and Tricare | Comment | EDI |
| Personal | Account | **Diagnosis** | Policy 1 | Policy 2 | Policy 3 |

Save

Principal Diagnosis: 034.0 ▼ 🔎 Strep Throat   POA ☐   Cancel

Default Diagnosis 2:

Code 1	Description
034.0	Strep Throat
052.9	Chicken Pox
075.0	Mononucleosis
250.01	IDDM Diabetes Mellitis
346.9	Headache-Migraine
401.9	Hypertension
422.9	Heart Disease
469.9	Upper Respiratory Infection

Default Diagnosis 3:

Default Diagnosis 4:

Help

Allergies and Notes

UB04...

gibility...

- Click on the Condition tab, and fill in the following information by selecting from drop-down lists or typing it.

Case: ADAJO000 Adams, Joan Q [Strep Throat]

| Personal | Account | Diagnosis | Policy 1 | Policy 2 | Policy 3 |
| **Condition** | Miscellaneous | Medicaid and Tricare | Comment | EDI |

Save

Injury/Illness/LMP Date: 9/17/2008   Date Similar Symptoms: ____   Cancel

Illness Indicator: Illness ▼   ☐ Same/Similar Symptoms

First Consultation Date: 9/17/2008 ▼   ☐ Employment Related

☐ Emergency   Help

Accident
Related To: ▼   State: ☐

Last X-Ray Date: ____ ▼

Death/Status

Nature Of: ▼   ____ ▼

UB04...

Dates
	From	To
Unable to Work:	9/18/2008	9/22/2008
Total Disability:		
Partial Disability:		
Hospitalization:		

Eligibility...

Workers' Compensation
Return To Work Indicator:
Normal ▼

Percent of Disability: ____

Last Worked Date: ____ ▼

☐ Pregnant

Estimated Date of Birth: ____ ▼

Date Assumed Care: ____ ▼

Date Relinquished Care: ____ ▼

Patient Information
Name: Adams, Joan Q.
Address: 540 Broadway
New York, NY
10025

Home Phone: (212)555-9999
Work Phone:
Cell Phone:
Date of Birth: 5/25/1946

Case
▼ 🔎

- Click on the Policy 1 tab, and enter the following:

Case: ADAJO000 Adams, Joan Q [Strep Throat]

Condition	Miscellaneous	Medicaid and Tricare	Comment	EDI

Personal	Account	Diagnosis	**Policy 1**	Policy 2	Policy 3

Insurance 1: AET00 ▼ 🔍 Aetna

Policy Holder 1: ADAJO000 ▼ 🔍 Adams, Joan Q

Relationship to Insured: Self ▼

Policy Number: 1111111111

Group Number: 02001

Policy Dates
Start: 9/1/2000 ▼
End: ▼

Claim Number:

☐ Assignment of Benefits/Accept Assignment   Deductible Met: ☐

☐ Capitated Plan   Annual Deductible: 500.00

Copayment Amount: 10.00

Treatment Authorization:

Document Control Number:

Insurance Coverage Percents by Service Classification   A: 80

Patient Information
Name: Adams, Joan Q.
Address: 540 Broadway
New York, NY
10025

Home Phone: (212)555-9999
Work Phone:
Cell Phone:
Date of Birth: 5/25/1946

[Buttons: Save, Cancel, Help, UB04..., Eligibility...]

Case: ▼ 🔍

- Click on the Save button on the upper right corner of the screen.

Transaction Entry and Claim Management

To enter transactions using MediSoft Advanced, click on the Transactions icon or pull down the Activities menu and select Enter Transactions.

Transaction Entry

Chart: ▼ 🔍

Case: ▼ 🔍

Last Payment Date:
Last Payment Amount:
Last Visit Date:
Visit: of
Global Coverage Until:

Charges:

Policy 1	Policy 2	Policy 3	Patient

0-30	31-60	61-90	91+

Total: TNB:

Policy Copay: OA:
Annual Deductible: YTD:

Charges:
Adjustments:
Subtotal:
Payment:
Balance:

Account Total:

Totals Charge

●	Principal Procedure	Chart Number	Case Number	Entry Number	Claim Number	Date From	Date To	Document Number	Description	Attending Provide
▶	☐									

Fill in the following dialog box by selecting Joan Adams's chart number and selecting the rest of the information from the drop-down list. Fill in the payment information in the bottom part of the window. Remember to click the Apply Command button. Create and send the claim to her insurance.

Enter a new case for Miriam Cohen. On September 24, 2008, Miriam attempted to remove an air conditioner and suffered severe back spasms. She was given an emergency appointment with Dr. Malloy. Click on the Office Hours icon on the toolbar. Double-click the space next to 8:15a, and enter the following:

Close Office Hours. Click on the Patient List icon or pull down the Lists menu and select Patients/Guarantors and Cases. Click on Miriam Cohen, and click the Case option button. Click New and fill in the following information on the Personal tab:

Click on the Policy 1 tab, and enter the following:

Medisoft Demo - Dr Phiyllis Malloy - [Case: COHMI000 Cohen, Miriam B [Back Spasm]]

File   Edit   Activities   Lists   Reports   Tools   Window   Services   Help

Condition | Miscellaneous | Medicaid and Tricare | Comment | EDI
Personal | Account | Diagnosis | **Policy 1** | Policy 2 | Policy 3

Insurance 1: BLU00   Blue Cross/Blue Shield

Policy Holder 1: COHMI000   Cohen, Miriam B

Relationship to Insured: Self

Policy Number: 3

Group Number: 4

Policy Dates
Start: 2/5/2008
End:

Claim Number:

☐ Assignment of Benefits/Accept Assignment   Deductible Met: ☐
☐ Capitated Plan   Annual Deductible: 750.00
                                                Copayment Amount: 0.00

Treatment Authorization: |

Document Control Number:

Insurance Coverage
Percents by Service   A: 80
Classification

Click the Account tab, and make sure PM is listed as the provider. Click the Diagnosis tab and select Low Back Pain from the principal diagnosis drop-down list. Click the Condition tab, and select Illness from the Illness Indicator drop-down list. Enter the first consultation date as 9/24/2008, and the dates unable to work as 9/23/2008 to 9/29/2008. Save your changes and close the Patient List window.

To enter a transaction for Miriam Cohen, click on the Transaction icon or pull down the Activities menu and choose Enter Transactions. Select Miriam Cohen's chart number from the drop-down list; select the case for back spasm. Make sure the Charge tab is selected. Enter *low back pain* as the description, and from the Procedure drop-down list, select Office Visit, Est Patient. The amount indicated as a charge should be $125.00. This amount should be automatically filled in once the correct procedure is selected. After the charge has been entered, proceed to enter a cash payment from Miriam Cohen of $50.00 and apply the payment to the charge. Click Save Transaction.

Print a receipt for her by clicking the Print Receipt button. Click Save Transaction.

Next we will create a claim to send to her insurance company. Her insurance must be billed for the remainder of the payment. You can create a claim for her either from the transaction screen by clicking on Print Claim or from Claim Management. MediSoft will not allow the creation of duplicate claims. Click Print Claim, select Paper as the billing method, and click OK. Choose Laser CMS (Primary) W/Form, and click Start to preview the report on the screen. You will see the claim on the screen. When you close out of this screen, you will receive a message that one claim has been created. If you need to edit the claim, highlight the claim in the Claim Management window and click Edit. You can check the status of your claims at the Claim Management window (pull down the Activities menu and select Claim Management). The claim is ready to send.

You can change the status to Sent by highlighting the claim, clicking on the Change Status button, and changing the status from Ready to Send. (In addition, you can change the status to Rejected, Challenged, and others).

Close the Claim Management window.

Next assume for the purposes of this exercise that the $75.00 payment is received immediately from Blue Cross/Blue Shield. Apply it to Miriam's account.

When you finish, your screen should look like this:

To enter the next case, you must first add the diagnosis code for a routine health screen exam to your diagnosis list. Pull down the List menu and select Diagnosis Code. In the Diagnosis (New) window, enter the code V70.0 and the description as Exam Routine Health Screen. Save this record.

Enter a new case for Karen Wang. Click on the Personal tab of the New Case dialog box and fill in the following information:

Click on the Diagnosis tab, and in the first drop-down list, select Exam Routine Health Screen as the principal diagnosis.

Click on the Policy 1 tab, and fill in the following information:

Insurance 1:	CIG00 ▼ 🔎 Cigna
Policy Holder 1:	WANKA000 ▼ 🔎 Wang, Karen
Relationship to Insured:	Self ▼
Policy Number:	6
Group Number:	7
Policy Dates Start:	7/9/2007 ▼
End:	▼
Claim Number:	
☐ Assignment of Benefits/Accept Assignment	Deductible Met: ☐
☐ Capitated Plan	Annual Deductible: 0.00
	Copayment Amount: 0.00
Treatment Authorization:	
Document Control Number:	
Insurance Coverage Percents by Service Classification	A: 80

Remember to save the information. (Keep in mind, you can either save as you enter the information under each tab or you can wait until all the information in each tab area is completed. Then select save.)

Ms. Wang has an appointment for an exam routine health screen, for which the charge is $45.00. Karen has insurance that pays $35.00. Create a claim for Karen Wang. Assume for the purpose of this exercise that CIGNA sends the $35.00 immediately. Apply the payment to Ms. Wang's account. The $10.00 is written off by the practice and is an adjustment to Karen's account. To enter transactions for Karen Wang, pull down the Activities menu and select Enter Transactions. You are entering three transactions: one for the charge of $45.00, a second for the CIGNA payment of $35.00, and a third for the CIGNA write-off of $10.00.

Medisoft Demo - Dr Phiyllis Malloy - [Transaction Entry]

File Edit Activities Lists Reports Tools Window Services Help

Chart: WANKA000   Wang, Karen (5/3/1970)

Case: 3   General Health Screen Panel

	Cigna	Patient					Charges:	$45.00
						Adjustments:	-$10.00
	0-30	31-60	61-90	91+		Subtotal:	$35.00
	0.00	$0.00	$0.00	$0.00		Payment:	-$35.00
	Total: $0.00					Balance:	$0.00

Last Payment Date: 9/24/2008
Last Payment Amount: -$35.00
Last Visit Date:
Visit: 0 of 0
Charges: Global Coverage Until:

Policy Copay: 0.00   OA:
Annual Deductible: 0.00 YTD: $0.00

Account Total: $0.00

	Principal Procedure	Chart Number	Case Number	Entry Number	Claim Number	Date From	Date To	Document Number	Description
▶	✔	WANKA000	3	6	0	9/24/2008	9/24/2008	0809240000	Exam ruotine health screen

New   Delete   MultiLink   Note

Payments, Adjustments, And Comments:

	Date	Pay/Adj Code	Who Paid	Description	Provider	Amount	Check Number	Unapplied
	9/24/2008	CIG	Cigna -Primary	Cigna Payment	PM	-35.00		$0.00
▶	9/24/2008	CIGWROFF	Cigna -Primary	Cigna Write-off	PM	-10.00		$0.00

To review, a claim is a bill sent to an insurance carrier. Claim management involves editing, sorting, and sending out claims on paper or electronically.

You have created claims for Miriam Cohen and Karen Wang. You can check the status of all your claims in the Claim Management window. If the list were too long and included claims that were no longer needed, you could delete claims in this window.

Printing Reports

Every morning the practice prints out a superbill (encounter form) for each patient with an appointment. Make a fifteen-minute appointment today for Joan Q. Adams at 9:00 AM for a general health screen. Print her superbill by doing the following: In the MediSoft program (not Office Hours), pull down the Reports menu and select Superbills. In the dialog box that opens, click OK.

In the Print Report Where? dialog box, click Start.

Select Joan Q. Adams's chart number in the Chart Number Range drop-down list in the Data Selection Questions dialog box. Delete any other information in the remaining boxes.

Click OK and the following superbill will appear:

Preview Report — Goto Page: 1 — 1 of 1

1001	Dr. Phiyllis Malloy	Date: 9/25/2008
	125 West 100th Street	
	New York, NY 10025	
	(212)555-5555	

ADAJO000	Adams, Joan Q	9/25/2008	9:00:00 AM

EXAM

EXAM	FEE
New Patient	
Problem Focused	99201
Expanded Problem, Focused	99202
Detailed	99203
Comprehensive	99204
Comprehrnsive/High Complex	99204
Initial Visit/Procedure	99025
Well Exam Infant (up to 12 mos.)	99318
Well Exam 1 - 4 yrs.	99382
Well Exam 5 - 11 yrs.	99383
Well Exam 12 - 17 yrs.	99384
Well Exam 18 - 39 yrs.	99385
Well Exam 40 - 64 yrs.	99386
Established Patient	
Minimum	99211
Problem Focused	99212
Expanded Problem Focused	99213
Detailed	99214
Comprehensive/High Complex	99215
Well Exam Infant(up to 12 mos.)	99391
Well exam 1 - 4 yrs.	99392
Well Exam 5 - 11 yrs.	99393
Well Exam 12 - 17 yrs.	99394
Well Exam 18 - 39 yrs.	99395
Well Exam 40 - 64 yrs.	99396
Obstetrics	
Total OB Care	59400
Obstetrical Visit	99212
Injections	
Administration Sub. / IM	90782
Drug	
Dosage	
Allegery	95155

PROCEDURES

PROCEDURES	FEE
Anoscopy	46600
Arthrocentesis/Aspiration/Injection	
Small Joint	*20600
Interm Joint	*20605
Major Joint	*20610
Audiometry	92552
Cast Application	
Location Long Short	
Catherization	*53670
Circumcision	54150
Colposcopy	*57452
Colposcopy w/Biopsy	*57454
Cryosurgery Premalignant Lesion	
Location(s):	
Cryosurgery Warts	
Location(s):	
Curettement Lesion w/Biopsy	CTF
Curettement Lesion wo/Biopsy	
Single	*11050
2 - 4	*11051
> 4	*11052
Diaphram Fitting	*57170
Ear Irrigation	69210
ECG	93000
Endometrial Biopsy	*58100
Exc. Lesion w/Biopsy	CTF
w/o Biopsy	
Location Size	
Exc. Skin Tags (1 - 15)	*11200
Each Additional 10	*11201
Fracture Treatment	
Loc	
w/Reduc w/o Reduc	
Fracture Treatment F/U	99024
I & D Abscess Single/Simple	*10060

LABORATORY

LABORATORY	FEE	
Aerobic Culture	87070	
Amylase	82150	
B12	82607	
CBC & Diff	85025	
CHEM 20	80019	
Chlamydia Screen	86317	
Cholesterol	82465	
Digoxin	80162	
Electrolytes	80005	
Ferritin	82728	
Folate	82746	
GC Screen	87070	
Glucose	82947	
Glucose 1 HR	82950	
Glycosylated HGB (A1C)	83036	
HCT	85014	
HDL	83718	
Hep BSAG	86278	
Hepatitis Profile	80059	
HGB & HCT	85014	
HIV	86311	
Iron & TIBC	83540	83550
Kidney Profile	80007	
Lead	83655	
Liver Profile	82977	
Mono Test	86308	
Pap Smear	88155	
Pregnancy Test	84703	
Prenatal Profile	80055	
Pro Time	85610	
PSA	84153	
RPR	86592	
Sed. Rate	85651	
Stool Culture	87045	
Stool O & P	87177	

Prior to entering the new transaction for Ms. Adams's appointment, you must first enter a new case for this appointment. Click on Patient List icon or pull down the Lists menu then click on Patients/Guarantors and Cases. Select Joan Adams's name from the Patient List, make sure that Case (by the chart number drop-down list) is selected, and click the New Case button. The description is General Health Screen, and her diagnosis is Exam Routine Health Screen. Make sure that the physician PM is selected and that her insurance listed is Aetna. Save the case record. If you find that you did not enter all of the information or need to correct something on a patient's case, you can update unclosed cases by going back into the case file for the patient and selecting the correct case by using the drop-down list on the bottom right hand side of the screen.

Case Selection

Drop-down list

Once the case on Ms. Adams has been entered, then it is time to enter the new transactions. Enter two new transactions for Ms. Adams that reflect the charge of $45.00 and her cash copayment of $10.00. Remember to apply the payment and save the transaction.

Once the transactions are entered, you can create a walkout receipt to be handed to the patient as he or she is leaving the office. To create a walkout receipt, click Print Receipt. In the Open Report dialog box, select Walkout Receipt (All Transactions), and click OK.

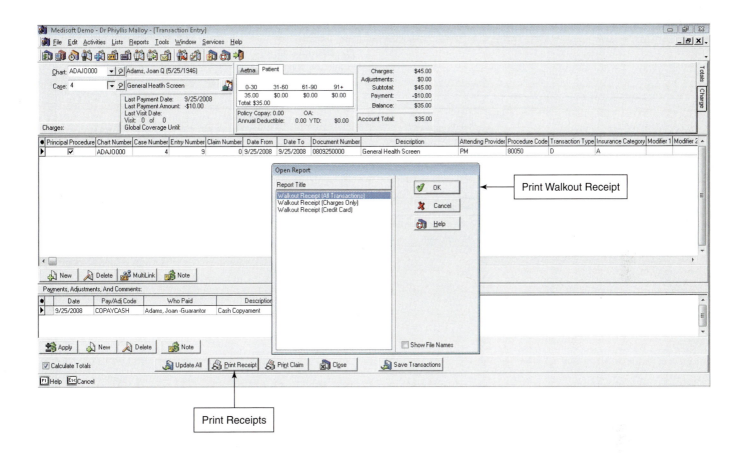

In the Print Where? dialog box, click Start. In the Data Selection Question dialog box, enter the date of the office visit and click OK. The following will appear:

To create a new insurance claim (the bill sent to the insurance carrier), click the Print Claim button. Select the Laser CMS (Primary) W/Form, select Preview the Report on the Screen, select Joan Q. Adams's chart number, and click OK.

To print a patient statement for Ms. Adams, pull down the Reports menu and select Patient Statements. On the Report Title window, select Patient Statement and click OK. Select View the Report on the Screen and click Start. Select Joan Q. Adams's chart number in the drop-down list and click OK. The following statement will appear:

Dr. Phiyllis Malloy
Patient Day Sheet
September 25, 2008
ALL

Entry	Date	Document	POS	Description	Provider	Code	Modifiers	Amount
ADAJO000 Adams, Joan Q								
11	9/25/2008	0809250000	11	General Health Screen	PM	80050		45.00
12	9/25/2008	0809250000	11	Cash Copayment	PM	COPAYCAS1		-10.00

Patient's Charges	Patient's Receipts	Insurance Receipts	Adjustments	Patient Balance
$45.00	-$10.00	$0.00	$0.00	$35.00

A patient day sheet is a report that lists each patient's name, chart number, and transactions for a particular day. To print a patient day sheet, pull down the Reports menu and select Day Sheets. Choose Patient Day Sheet. On the next screen, leave all the information as is, and select Preview Report. The following report will be generated.

Patient: Joan Q. Adams		Chart #: ADAJO000			
Case Description: Strep Throat		Date of Last Payment: 9/25/2008	Amount:	-10.00	
9/17/2008	0809240000	Culture, Strep Throat		1	15.00
9/17/2008	0809240000	Cash Payment - Thanks		1	-15.00
Patient: Joan Q. Adams		Chart #: ADAJO000			
Case Description: General Heatlh Sc	Date of Last Payment: 9/25/2008		Amount:	-10.00	
9/25/2008	0809250000	General Health Screen Panel		4	45.00
9/25/2008	0809250000	Cash Copayment		4	-10.00

Total Charges	Total Payments	Total Adjustments	**Balance Due**
$60.00	-$25.00	$0.00	**35.00**

Summary

- MediSoft allows the office worker in a health-care environment to enter the information necessary to establish a database for a new practice. This includes practice, provider, insurance, address, and diagnosis information.
- Diagnosis codes, billing, procedure, payment, and adjustment codes can also be entered in tables.
- MediSoft is primarily an accounting program. Transactions (charges, payments, and adjustments) can be entered and payments applied. Claims can be created and sent to insurance carriers.
- Several reports can be generated, including a superbill (encounter form), patient statements, and patient day sheets.

CHAPTER ELEVEN

UTILITIES

THIS CHAPTER IS FOR INFORMATION ONLY. YOU <u>CANNOT</u> USE MEDISOFT'S FILE MAINTENANCE AND BACKUP UTILITIES IN A CLASSROOM SETTING.

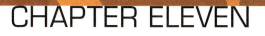

Chapter Outline

- File Maintenance
- Backup Utility
- Summary
- Review Exercises

Learning Objectives

Upon completion of this chapter, the student will be aware of MediSoft's file maintenance and backup utilities.

Key Terms

Back Up
Packing Data
Purging Data

Rebuilding Indexes
Recalculating Balances

File Maintenance

If you were in a working environment and wanted to access MediSoft's utility programs, you would pull down the File menu and choose File Maintenance.

The following screen is displayed:

File Maintenance		
Purge Data	Recalculate Balances	
Rebuild Indexes	Pack Data	

The list below represents the data files used by this program. Place a check mark by each file for which you would like to verify and rebuild. Depending on the size of the file, this process may take a LONG time.

Press START to begin the process.

☐ Address	☐ Patient	☐ Collection List
☐ Office Hours Files	☐ Provider	☐ Security Groups
☐ Case	☐ Referring Provider	☐ Work Flow Administration
☐ Claim	☐ Procedure Code	☐ Claims Manager
☐ Diagnosis	☐ Transaction	☐ Unprocessed Transactions
☐ Electronic Claim Receiver	☐ Recall	
☐ Insurance Carrier	☐ Resource	
☐ MultiLink Codes	☐ Billing Codes	
☐ Custom Data	☐ Allowed Amount	
☐ Pin Matrix	☐ Treatment Plan	
☐ Deposit	☐ Superbill Tracking	
☐ Permissions	☐ Zip Code	
☐ Multimedia	☐ Contact Log	
☐ Eligibility	☐ Defaults	
☐ Credit Card		
☐ Statement		

☐ All Files

Start · Cancel · Help

Rebuilding indexes checks the structure of records; it does not change or delete any data.

Packing data compresses data. MediSoft keeps the record structure even after its contents have been deleted. Packing data gets rid of the empty records.

Purging data permanently deletes patients who no longer visit the practice. It can also be used to delete cases, appointments, claims, and audit data. Extreme care should be used when deleting.

Recalculating balances updates balances so they reflect the newest entries.

Backup Utility

It is necessary to back up (put copies of files onto some form of removable media) all data processed on a computer. Data can be lost due to computer failure, natural disaster, theft, or human error. If you were in an office, you would need to set up a schedule to back up your data. Daily backups to CDs or flash drives and weekly backups to a higher-capacity medium such as an external hard drive can protect your data; you lose only what is entered or edited after the last backup. If your computer crashes, you may need to reinstall MediSoft, but at least your data will be safe; you can restore it using your backup. MediSoft provides a backup utility, which can be used in a real work environment; to access it, pull down the File menu and select Backup Data. If your computer crashes, you may need to reinstall MediSoft and restore the data using your backup medium. However, you will lose all data entered after your last backup. A word of caution: When you back up a practice's database files, only the active database is being backed up. Each practice's database must be backed up separately.

Summary

- MediSoft provides the user in an office environment with utilities to help maintain files and back up data.

Review Exercises

Define the Following Terms:

Packing data

Purging data

Rebuilding indexes

Recalculating balances

Discuss the Following:

Why is it necessary to backup your data? In your answer refer to the various threats to computer systems and data.

UB-04 CLAIMS

Appendix Outline

- UB-04 Claims Overview
- Turning on the UB-04 Fields
- Establishing a New Practice
- Entering Patient Information
- Entering Insurance Carrier
- Entering Diagnosis Codes
- Entering Procedure Code
- Entering Cases
- Additional Resources on the UB-04
- Summary

Learning Objectives

Although most of you will not submit UB-04 claims using MediSoft, since MediSoft offers this function, this appendix provides instruction on how a UB-04 claim is processed using MediSoft. Upon completion of this appendix, the student will understand more about the process of sending UB-04 claims using MediSoft and will be able to perform the following tasks:

- Enable UB-04 fields
- Establish a new practice
- Enter new patient information
- Enter diagnosis codes
- Enter insurance carrier information
- Enter diagnosis and procedure codes
- Enter a new case for an existing patient
- Enter information into UB-04 fields

UB-04 Claims Overview

A new feature of MediSoft version 14 is the ability to provide UB-04 claims support. UB-04 claims are those claims processed by institutional providers such as hospitals and skilled nursing facilities. When using MediSoft, UB-04 fields can be enabled and UB-04 claims can be processed. Once you have entered data in the appropriate UB-04 fields, you can enter transactions and create and print a UB-04 claim.

Turning on the UB-04 Fields

To begin using the UB-04 function in MediSoft, you must first enable UB-04 fields. Because not all offices process these types of claims, this field is turned off by default. If your facility requires the processing of UB-04 claims, then it is important to ensure that the UB-04 fields are enabled. This is done by clicking on File, Program Options, Data Entry, and ensuring that the Suppress UB-04 Fields option is unchecked.

Once the UB-04 fields have been turned on, they will appear in various places when using the MediSoft program.

Establishing a New Practice

First let's establish a new practice.

- Pull down the File menu, and click New Practice.
- Add the following information and indicate the data path:

- Click the Create button to save your entry.
- In the next window, complete the following information and save the record.

Francis J. McCaslin is a provider who works at University Medical Center. Add Dr. McCaslin as a provider in the new practice you just established and click Save.

Once your new provider information has been entered, pull up your Provider List to check your information.

● To add the Physician's PIN, highlight the physician you just entered, press Edit, select the PIN tab, then select the insurance for which the PIN should be entered.

● Save the record.

Entering Patient Information

Let's create a new patient for our UB-04 claim:

- To enter patient data, click the Patient List icon or pull down the Lists menu and choose Patients/Guarantors and Cases.
- Click New.
- Enter the following information in the Name, Address page of the dialog box:

- Do not enter a chart number. MediSoft will automatically enter it for you when you save the record.
- Click the Other Information tab, and fill it in as follows:

Medisoft Demo - University Medical Center - [Address: Olive's Garden]

File   Edit   Activities   Lists   Reports   Tools   Window   Services   Help

Code: [   ]   If the Code is left blank, the program will assign one.

Name: Olive's Garden

Street: 10305 Gateway West

City: New York   State: NY

Zip Code: 10025

Type: Employer

Phone: (212)555-2611   Extension: [   ]

Fax Phone: [   ]

Cell Phone: [   ]

Office: [   ]

Contact: [   ]

E-Mail: [   ]

ID: [   ]

Identifier: [   ]

Entity ID: [   ]   Purchased Services: ☐

Mammography Certification: [   ]

Extra 1: [   ]   Extra 2: [   ]

To enter the employer information, place your cursor in the Employer area and right-click, select New Employer from the menu. Enter the information and click Save.

You will be brought back to the Patient List. Close this window.

Entering Insurance Carrier

You also need to enter the insurance carrier.

- Pull down the Lists menu, and choose Insurance then Carriers.
- In the dialog box that opens, click New.

● Add the following information:

Insurance Carrier: BCBS HMO

Address | Options | EDI/Eligibility | Codes | PINs

Code: [   ]   If the Code is left blank, the program will assign one.   ☐ Inactive

Name: BCBS HMO
Street: 6933 Coit
[   ]
City: New York   State: NY
Zip Code: 10025

Phone: (212)432-1234   Extension: 1234
Fax: [   ]
Contact: [   ]
Practice ID: [   ]

Save
Cancel
Help

- Click the Options tab, and enter the following information:

- Save the record and MediSoft assigns a code.

Entering Diagnosis Codes

You now need to add the diagnosis of Hepatorenal Syndrome. Do the following:

- Click on the Dx (diagnosis) icon or pull down Lists menu and choose Diagnosis Codes. Diagnosis codes are added one at a time.
- Click New and fill in the following information:
  - Code 1   572.4
  - Description   Hepatorenal Syndrome

- Save the record.

Entering Procedure Code

For the purpose of this exercise, the procedure code of 78205 must be entered.

- Click on the CPT icon or pull down the Lists menu and select Procedure, Payment, and Adjustment list. Click New. A two-tabbed dialog box is displayed. You need to fill in information on each page of the dialog box.
- Enter 78205 as Code 1.
- Enter Radioisotope Scan of the Liver as the Description.
- Enter Procedure Charge as the code type (select it using the code type drop-down list).
- The Type of Service should be 5. The type of service identifies the service as a charge, payment, adjustment, or procedure.
- Enter 0 as Time to Do Procedure.

- Click on the Amounts tab and enter $756.50 as Charge Amount A. This is the price the facility charges for the service.
- Save the record.

Entering Cases

To enter a new case for Alyssa M. Smith, do the following:

- Pull down the Lists menu, and select Patients/Guarantors and Cases.
- Click on Alyssa M. Smith, and click the Case option button.
- Click New Case.
- Click on the Personal tab.

Fill in the description, the marital status, and the student status as shown below:

The rest of the information has already been entered or provided by MediSoft.

- Click on the Account tab, and ensure Dr. McCaslin is selected.
- Click on the Diagnosis tab, and select Hepatorenal Syndrome from the drop-down list.
- Click on the Condition tab, and select Illness from the drop-down list under Illness Indicator.
- Click on the Policy 1 tab, and enter the following:

Medisoft Demo - University Medical Center - [Case: SMIAL000 Smith, Alyssa M]

File Edit Activities Lists Reports Tools Window Services Help

Condition | Miscellaneous | Medicaid and Tricare | Comment | EDI
Personal | Account | Diagnosis | **Policy 1** | Policy 2 | Policy 3

Insurance 1: BCB00 ▼ ⌕ BCBS HMO

Policy Holder 1: SMIAL000 ▼ ⌕ Smith, Alyssa M

Relationship to Insured: Self ▼

Policy Number: ZGY563885691

Group Number: 00063952

Policy Dates
Start: 5/7/2007 ▼
End: ▼

Claim Number:

☑ Assignment of Benefits/Accept Assignment   Deductible Met: ☐
☐ Capitated Plan   Annual Deductible: 0.00
                                                 Copayment Amount: 0.00

Treatment Authorization: 693358924
Document Control Number: 36249967

Insurance Coverage   A: 80
Percents by Service
Classification

- To fill out the UB-04 information, click on the UB-04 button on the far right-hand side of the screen.
- Complete FL4 through FL41 as shown here:

Note that for this example, some of the fields are not used.

- When done with FL4 through FL41, click on the tab to view fields FL67 through FL81. For this example, these fields are not used.
- Click on the Save button in the upper right corner of the screen.

Additional Resources on the UB-04

For additional information on the UB-04, the following resources are helpful:

National Uniform Billing Committee (the organization that maintains the UB-04): www.nubc.org

Centers for Medicare and Medicaid: www.cms.hhs.gov. Once you are at this site, click on the Outreach & Education tab and under Medicare Learning Network (MLN), select MLN Educational Web Guides. Under Web-Based Training Courses, there is a free online course on the UB-04.

For further information on the UB-04 in your region, you can also check out the site for your regional Medicare contractor and Blue Cross plan.

Summary

- MediSoft version 14 has added UB-04 claims support.
- UB-04 claims are those claims processed by institutional providers such as hospitals and skilled nursing facilities.
- To begin using the UB-04 function, you must first ensure that the UB-04 fields are enabled.
- Once you have entered data in the appropriate UB-04 fields, you can enter transactions on a patient and create and print a UB-04 claim.

INTRODUCTION TO COMPUTERS AND COMPUTER LITERACY

Appendix Outline

- Computer Literacy
- What Is a Computer?
- Data Representation
- Computer Hardware
  - Input Devices
  - Processing Hardware and Memory
  - Output Devices
  - Secondary Storage Devices
- Software
  - System Software
  - Applications Software
- Summary
- Resources for Information on the Use of Computers

Learning Objectives

Upon completion of this appendix, the student will:

- Be able to define the terms *computer literacy* and *computer*.
- Be able to discuss how the computer represents data.
- Know the difference between computer hardware and software.
- Comprehend the data processing cycle.

Key Terms

Applications Software

Arithmetic-Logic Unit (ALU)

Automatic Recalculation

Binary Digit

Bit

Boot

Bus

Byte

Cache

Carpal Tunnel Syndrome

CD-R (Compact Disk-Recordable)

CD-ROM (Compact Disk with Read-Only Memory)

CD-RW (Compact Disk-Rewriteable)

Central Processing Unit (CPU)

Computer

Computer Literacy

Control Unit (CU)

Data

Database Management
    Software (DBMS)

Digital Camera

Digitize

Direct Access

Direct-Entry Devices

Disk Drive

Diskette

Dot-Matrix Printer

DVD

Electronic Spreadsheet

Embedded Computer

Ergonomics

Fax Machine

Graphical User Interface (GUI)

Hard Copy

Hard Disk

Hardware

Head Crash

Impact Printer

Information

Ink-Jet Printer

Input Device

Internet

Keyboard

Kurzweil Scanner

Laser Printer

Line-of-Sight System

Magnetic Disk

Magnetic Ink Character
    Recognition (MICR)

Magnetic Stripe

Magnetic Tape

Mainframe

Megahertz

Memory

Microcomputer

Monitor

Motherboard

Nonimpact Printer

Operating System (OS)

Optical Card

Optical Character Recognition
    (OCR)

Optical Disk

Optical Mark Recognition
    (OMR)

Output Device

Pen-Based System

Personal Computer (PC)

Plotter

Pointing Device

Printer

Processing Hardware

Processing Unit

Processor

Program

QWERTY

Random-Access Memory
    (RAM)

Read-Only Memory (ROM)

Read/Write Head

Scanning Device

Secondary Storage Device

Secondary Storage Medium

Sensor

Sequential Access Storage
    Medium

Smart Card

Soft Copy

Software

Speech Input System

Speech Output System

Supercomputer

System Clock

System Software

System Unit

Tape

User

User Interface

Utility Program

Word Processing Software

Word Size

World Wide Web

Computer Literacy

A general knowledge of computers and their uses in any career or field, particularly health care, is essential.

Computer literacy refers to knowledge of how to use computer information technology. The details of computer literacy are continually changing as computers and their uses change. A computer-literate person today knows how to use a computer in his own field to make tasks easier and to complete them more efficiently, has a vocabulary to discuss computers intelligently, and understands in a broad fashion what a computer is and what it can do. Today, unlike several years ago, computer literacy involves knowledge of the **Internet** and the **World Wide Web** and the ability to take advantage of these resources. Being computer literate does not mean you can build, fix, or program a computer. Familiarity with computers and the Internet is crucial in any field, including health care and its delivery. As in other fields, the basic tasks of gathering, allocating, controlling, and retrieving information are the same.

Although very few people question the necessity of learning about computers, some are still fearful of this technology. Knowledge is the best way to overcome this anxiety. It is definitely worth making the effort, since in every discipline, computers are playing a larger and more important role, and almost any employed person will have to be a competent computer **user**. This is particularly true in the field of health care and medical office management, where the ability to learn to use new programs specifically geared to medical office management can mean the difference between employment and unemployment.

What Is a Computer?

A **computer** is an electronic device that can accept **data** (raw facts) as input and process, manipulate, or alter them in some way to produce useful **information** as output. A computer processes data by following step-by-step instructions called a program. The program, the data, and the information need to be stored temporarily in memory while processing is going on and permanently on a secondary storage device for future use. Computers are accurate, fast, and reliable. Computers can be classified according to their size and power. However, every computer performs similar functions.

Classification of Computers by Size and Power

Supercomputer	The supercomputer is the fastest, most powerful computer available at any time. Supercomputers are used for scientific purposes, such as to simulate actual events to make prediction possible. For instance, supercomputers are used to forecast the weather, to see what would happen to a driver in a car crash, and to estimate the structure of a virus.
Mainframe	The mainframe is smaller than the supercomputer and is a multiuser system with many terminals using the power of one computer in what is called a timesharing environment. Unlike the supercomputer, the mainframe is used for business purposes, for repetitive tasks such as generating a payroll or processing insurance claims.
Microcomputer or Personal Computer (PC)	The PC is a single-user computer. They come in different sizes, from a small notebook to a powerful workstation. Microcomputers can be networked, making the information and programs available on one PC available to all on the network. When linked to the Internet, a microcomputer puts the world at your fingertips.
Embedded Computer	The embedded computer is a microprocessor that does one thing, such as regulate a heart pacemaker. It is embedded in the appliance and can be programmed to respond to changing conditions, for example, to help the heart only when help is needed.

Computer hardware includes all of the physical components of a computer. Each computer function that is performed has hardware associated with it. **Input devices** are used for entering data that is automatically converted into a form that the computer can process. A **processing unit** manipulates data. **Output devices** produce information useful to human beings. Memory provides temporary storage, and secondary storage devices allow for more permanent storage.

Data Representation

All data in a computer is represented by bits (binary digits). This includes characters, numbers, graphics, sound, animation, and so on. A bit is either a one or a zero.

Computer Hardware

Input Devices

Input hardware allows you to enter data that you understand and digitizes it or translates it into a form that the computer can process, that is, zeros and ones. Input devices can be divided into **keyboards** and **direct-entry devices**.

KEYBOARDS The keyboard with which you are familiar is called the **QWERTY** keyboard. It was invented during the nineteenth century for the mechanical typewriter. The arrangement of the keys was meant to slow typists down because if they typed too fast, the bars of type would jam. The keyboard most of us use is not conducive to fast data entry. It can also contribute to **carpal tunnel syndrome**, which is a painful compression of the median nerve in the wrist and the hand caused by repetitive motion. The field of **ergonomics** attempts to study the relationship between people and their work environment and to minimize work-related injuries by creating a safer and more efficient workplace.

The standard QWERTY keyboard contains several kinds of keys: the **alphanumeric** keyboard (letters and numbers) and special symbol keys (e.g., @, &, *, etc.). The Enter key is used to end a paragraph and enter commands; special **function keys** perform different tasks depending on the software you are using. When you press any key on the keyboard, it is immediately translated into machine language, a series of electronic pulses that the computer can process.

DIRECT-ENTRY DEVICES Direct-entry devices include **pointing devices**, such as a mouse, trackball, touch screen, and various kinds of pen-based input. **Pen-based systems** recognize handwriting. They are used in some hospitals to enter comments on a patient's chart. **Scanning devices** translate images into digital form by shining light on the image and measuring the reflection. Scanning devices include the bar-code scanner found in supermarkets; **optical mark recognition (OMR)**, which can sense a mark by a number 2 pencil on a Scantron grading sheet; **optical character recognition (OCR)**, which reads printed characters; and the **Kurzweil scanner**, which reads printed material aloud and is useful to those with impaired vision.

An early scanning device used in the banking industry reads the numbers printed on checks in magnetic ink. **Magnetic ink character recognition (MICR)** recognizes a small character set and is used almost exclusively by banks.

A **fax machine** is also a scanning device. It scans the text or image and converts it to electronic signals that are sent over phone lines; the receiving fax machine converts it back into text and images. A fax machine can scan whole pages of graphics and text and digitize them so the computer can process them. Once scanned, you can treat the text in the same way as text you typed.

Various types of cards are also used as input devices. The **magnetic stripe** on the back of your charge card or ATM card contains data, such as your account number, in a form a computer can read. A **smart card** looks like a regular credit card but contains a microprocessor chip and memory. It can do some processing and hold about thirty pages worth of data. Smart cards are used as debit cards. An **optical card** holds about two thousand pages of data. An optical card could be used to hold your whole medical history, including test results and X-rays. Small enough to carry in your wallet, the information on the optical card would be immediately available if you were hospitalized in an emergency.

Speech input systems began as adaptive technology to help people with vision impairments and people who could not use a keyboard. They allow the user to talk to the computer; the computer would then digitize the spoken words. A speech recognition system contains a dictionary of digital patterns of words. You say a word, and the system digitizes it and compares it to the words in its dictionary. Speech recognition systems have to be trained to recognize your speech; the more you talk to it, the more it understands your speech.

A computer uses a **digital camera** to digitize images and stores them. The computer sees by having the camera take a picture of an object. The digitized image of this object is then compared with the images in storage. This may be used to develop special glasses for Alzheimer's patients so they can identify people and attach a name to the face.

A **sensor**, of particular interest to health professionals, is a device that collects data directly from the environment and sends the data to a computer. Sensors are used to collect patient information for clinical monitoring systems, including physiological, arrhythmia, pulmonary, and obstetrical/neonatal systems. They can detect the smallest change in temperature or any other physiological measurement.

The newest kind of input devices allow you to use your body as an input device. Biometrics are being used in security systems to protect data from unauthorized users. Fingerprints, hand-prints, and iris scans are being used to identify authorized users. Human biology input devices include line-of-sight and brain wave input. With **Line-of-sight systems** use a camera and computer to identify where the user is looking. If the user has limited use of her limbs, she can look at a letter for a certain amount of time and the line-of-sight system will process that as if she typed the letter on a keyboard. Brain wave input involves implanting a chip in a stroke victim who has lost the ability to communicate. The chip allows the individual to write sentences on a computer screen by thinking.

Processing Hardware and Memory

Once data is input into the computer, it is processed, that is, manipulated in some way. Located on the main circuit board **(motherboard)**, the **processor** or **system unit** contains the **central processing unit (CPU)** and **memory**. In a microcomputer the microprocessor is on a chip. In a larger computer, the processor might be on several circuit boards. The CPU has two parts: The **arithmetic-logic unit (ALU)** performs the arithmetic operations of adding and subtracting, multiplying, dividing, and raising to a power, as well as the logical operation of comparing. The **control unit (CU)** directs the operation of the computer in accordance with the program's instructions.

The CPU works closely with memory, the computer's temporary workspace. The instructions of the program being executed must be in memory for processing to take place. Memory also is located on the computer's main circuit board. The central processing unit fetches one instruction at a time from memory and processes it.

The part of memory where current work is temporarily stored during processing is called **random-access memory (RAM)**. RAM also is on chips. It is temporary, volatile memory, meaning its contents disappear when the power is turned off. The size of RAM is important since the program you are executing and the work you create must be able to fit in RAM. Remember that a **byte** is eight bits—about the space it takes to store one character.

A small part of RAM is called **cache** memory; it is a special, high-speed, temporary storage area that holds the most often-used instructions. Data and instructions are moved from cache memory or RAM to the CPU on electronic pathways called **buses**. The other part of memory (also on chips) is called **read-only memory (ROM)** or firmware. ROM is permanent and contains basic start-up instructions for the computer; you cannot change the contents of ROM.

Several factors determine the speed of a computer, including the amount of RAM, word size, and clock speed. The amount of RAM affects the speed of the computer. If RAM is not big enough to hold what you are working with, your work is slowed considerably. Computer processors are made to handle a certain number of bits as a unit at one time. This is called its **word size**. The bigger the word size, the faster the processor. Processors contain a **system clock**, a vibrating quartz crystal, and the speed of the vibrations controls the speed of the processor. In a PC, clock speed is measured in **megahertz** (MHz; 1 million cycles per second).

Output Devices

Once data is processed, output devices translate what the computer understands (bits) into a form human beings can understand. Output devices are divided into two basic categories: those that produce **hard copy**, such as **printers** and **plotters**, and those that produce **soft copy**, such as **monitors** and **speech output systems**.

Printers may be **impact printers**, where a print head actually strikes the paper, or **nonimpact**. **Dot-matrix printers** are impact printers that form characters and images with pins striking an inked ribbon. Inexpensive and noisy, dot-matrix printers do not produce excellent output. Today nonimpact printers are more common. **Ink-jet printers** form letters by spraying dots of ink on paper. Ink-jet printers produce excellent-quality text and graphics in black and white and color at a low cost. **Laser printers** produce the best output but are the most expensive. The technology used by laser printers is similar to that used by photocopiers. For specialized graphics output, plotters can be used. Plotters have a pen mounted in a chassis that moves it up and down and back and forth across a paper. The paper is also mounted on rollers that can move it back and forth. The combination of the pen moving and the paper moving are used to create maps and architectural drawings.

The most commonly used output device is a monitor. Screens differ in size, color, and in the clarity of the display. Soft copy is also produced by devices that output sound, music, and speech.

Secondary Storage Devices

The memory we have discussed so far is temporary or volatile. To **save** your work more permanently, you need secondary storage devices. **Magnetic disks** (**diskette** or **hard disk**), **magnetic tapes**, and **optical disks** are used as secondary storage media. Magnetic media store data and programs as magnetic spots or electromagnetic charges. Optical disks store data as pits and lands burned into a plastic disk.

To use a diskette, it is inserted into a **secondary storage device** such as a **disk drive**, which has a motor to spin the disk and an access arm with a **read/write head** to move across it. It is this read/write head that reads data from (makes a copy of the data to put in RAM) and writes data to (takes what is in RAM and puts it on the disk) the diskette. A hard disk is similar but includes several platters made of metal or glass, and is encased in a sealed unit to keep contaminants away from the disk surfaces. Data is recorded on both sides of the platters. Hard disks hold much more data than floppies—up to several gigabytes. Access time is much faster because they spin continuously at a much higher speed. A potential disadvantage of hard drives is the possibility of a **head crash**; the cushion of air between the read/write head and the disk is tiny, and the disk is spinning so fast that any contamination can cause the head to touch the disk and may destroy the data.

Optical disks use laser technology to store data as pits and lands (flat areas) on a disk. Instead of an access arm and read/write head, a high-power laser burns tiny pits in the surface, and another lower-power laser reads the surface, interpreting the pits and lands as zeros and ones. The pits are so small (three thousand pits take up only one centimeter) that an enormous amount of data can be stored on one optical disk.

There are several kinds of optical disk. The **CD-ROM (compact disk with read-only memory)** is the most common. A CD-ROM is created at a factory; you can buy it, put it in your CD-ROM drive, and read the contents into the memory of your PC. However, you cannot change the contents of the CD-ROM. Their immense storage capacity of 680 megabytes is roughly equivalent to 477 high-density 3.5″ diskettes, or about 250,000 pages. This volume makes them ideal for distributing books and encyclopedias.

A **CD-R (compact disk-recordable)** is sold as a blank disk on which the user can create his or her own CD-ROM. Once created, however, it cannot be changed. A **CD-RW (compact disk-rewriteable)** can be read from and written to—much like a diskette. **DVDs** (digital video or digital versatile disks) are optical disks with a storage capacity of 4.7 gigabytes. A super DVD can hold up to 17 gigabytes.

Some of the advantages of optical disks include their great capacity, low cost, and durability. An optical disk lasts longer than magnetic media.

The oldest form of secondary storage is magnetic tape. The difference between retrieving data from tape and disk of any kind is like the difference between listening to music on audiotape and compact disk. A disk allows **direct access** to any piece of information on that specific disk. Unlike a disk, a tape is a **sequential access storage medium**. To get to the five hundredth piece of information on a tape, you need to fast forward through the first 499. A tape cartridge is loaded into a drive where the tape passes under a read/write head. Magnetic tape comes in different widths and lengths. It is the slowest and cheapest medium but holds a great deal of data. Today it is used mainly for backing up disk storage.

Larger computers use external hard disks for secondary storage. The disks differ in the size of the platters, the number of platters, and the recording capacity.

Software

Software refers to the programs, that is, the step-by-step instructions that tell the hardware what to do. Without software, hardware is useless. Software falls into two general categories: system software and applications software.

System Software

System software consists of programs that help the computer manage its own resources. The most important piece of system software is the operating system. The operating system is a group of programs that manages the resources of the computer. It controls the hardware, manages basic input and output operations, keeps track of files saved on disk and in memory, and directs communication between the CPU and other pieces of hardware. It coordinates how other programs work with the hardware and with each other. Operating systems also provide the **user interface**, that is, the way the user communicates with the computer. For example, Windows provides a **graphical user interface**, pictures or icons that you click on with a mouse. When the computer is turned on, the operating system is booted or loaded into the computer's RAM. No other program can work until the operating system is booted. There are several operating systems for microcomputers, including DOS (disk operating system), Windows, UNIX, and Macintosh. Utility programs such as screen savers and backup software are also examples of system software.

Applications Software

Applications software allows you to apply computer technology to a task you need done. There are applications packages for many needs.

Word processing software allows you to enter text for a paper, report, letter, or memo. Once it is entered, it can be edited (corrected and improved) and formatted (changed in appearance). The size, style, and face of the type; margins; justification; line spacing; and tab stops can all be changed.

Electronic spreadsheets allow you to process numerical data. Organized into rows and columns intersecting to form cells, spreadsheets make doing arithmetic almost fun. You enter the values you want processed and the formula that tells the software how to process the values, and the answer appears. If you find you made a mistake entering a value, just change it, and the answer is **automatically recalculated**. Spreadsheet software also allows the creation of graphs. Spreadsheets have several health-care-related applications. The Food and Drug Administration uses giant spreadsheets to keep records of clinical trials. A spreadsheet program can help with anything that can be reduced to numbers, such as tracking the spread of a disease, a hospital's financial planning, and materials management.

Database management software (DBMS) allows you to manage large quantities of data in an organized fashion. Information in a database is organized in tables. The database management software makes it easy to enter, edit, sort, or organize data; search for data that meets a particular criterion; and retrieve the data. Once the structure of the table is defined and the data entered, the data never has to be typed again. Attractive reports can be generated easily by simply defining their structure—not retyping the data. MediSoft allows the user to create relational databases, which can link tables of doctors, patients, cases, insurance codes, allowed amounts, procedure codes, and diagnostic codes. All this information is necessary to run a medical office and generate accurate bills.

Summary

- Computer literacy refers to the ability to use computers in your field, to use the Internet, and to be able to discuss computers intelligently.
- A computer is an electronic device that accepts data as input then processes the data and displays (on screen or paper) information as output. Information, data, and programs can be saved temporarily or permanently. The computer operates under the control of programs stored in memory. All computers perform the four functions of input, process, storage, and output.
- Data is represented inside the computer by zeros and ones.
- Computer hardware refers to the parts of the computer you can see, including input and output devices, processing hardware, internal memory, and secondary storage devices.
- System software includes programs that perform basic functions for the computer. The operating system takes care of basic input and output, keeps track of files, and manages processor time. Applications software does a task for you: Word processing programs allow you to type text documents. Electronic spreadsheets make math quick and easy. Database management software helps you organize huge masses of data.

Resources for Information on the Use of Computers

Derek K. Miller. "How to Keep out of Trouble with Your E-mail: Rules and Etiquette for Using Internet Electronic Mail." www.penmachine.com/techie/emailtrouble_2003-07.html.

Sara Baase. *A Gift of Fire: Social, Legal, and Ethical Issues in Computing*, 3rd ed . Upper Saddle River, NJ: Prentice-Hall, 2008.

American Medical Informatics Association, www.amia.org/index.asp.

IEEE Computer Society, www.computer.org/portal/site/ieeecs/index.jsp.

C. Martin Harris, MD. "Handheld Computers in Medicine: The Future Is Not Here Yet." *Cleveland Clinical Journal of Medicine,* 68(10), www.ccjm.org/pdffiles/Harris-ed1001.pdf.

Healthcare Information and Management Systems Society, www.himss.org/ASP/index.asp.

Online Doctors USA, www.onlinedoctorsusa.com.

MDs Medical: Electronic Medical Records Software, www.mdsmedicalsoftware.com/index.php.

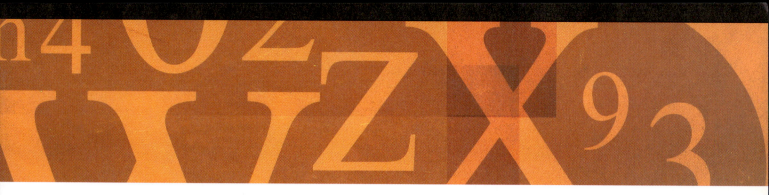

INDEX